A Little Of What You Fancy Does You Good

YOUR HEALTH IN LATER LIFE

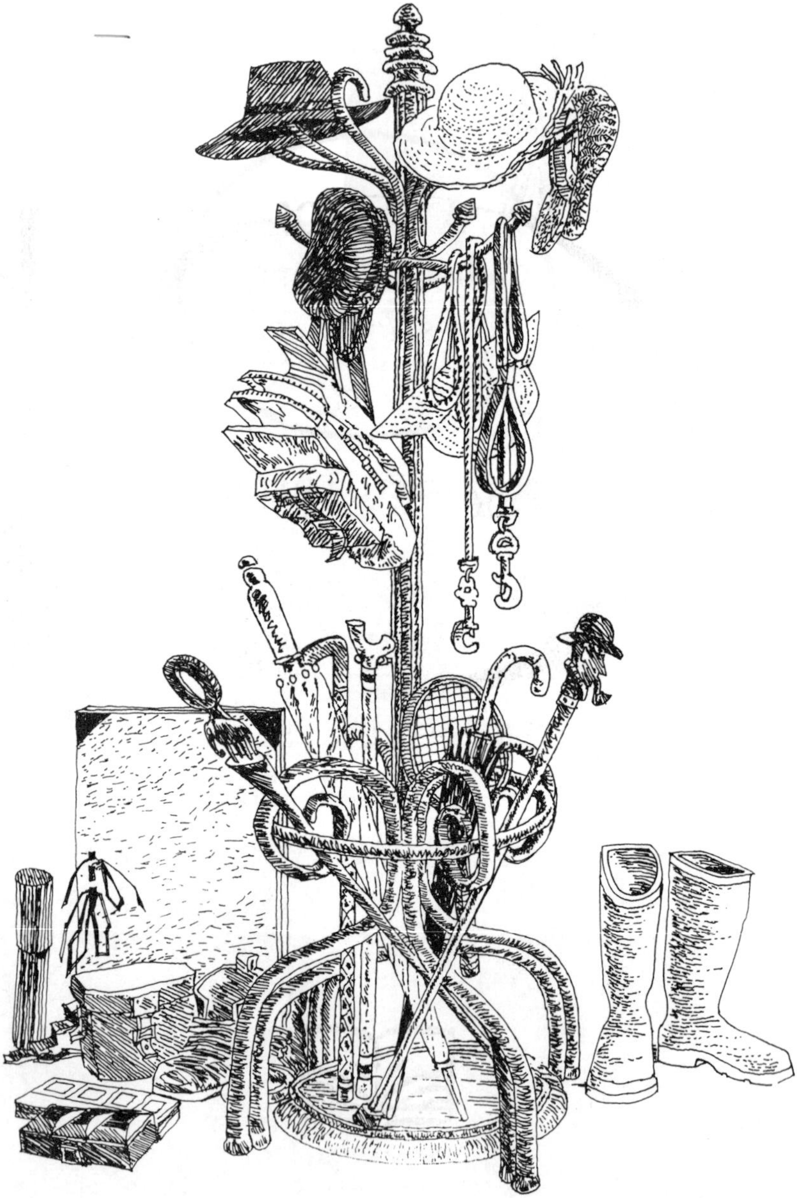

A Little Of What You Fancy Does You Good

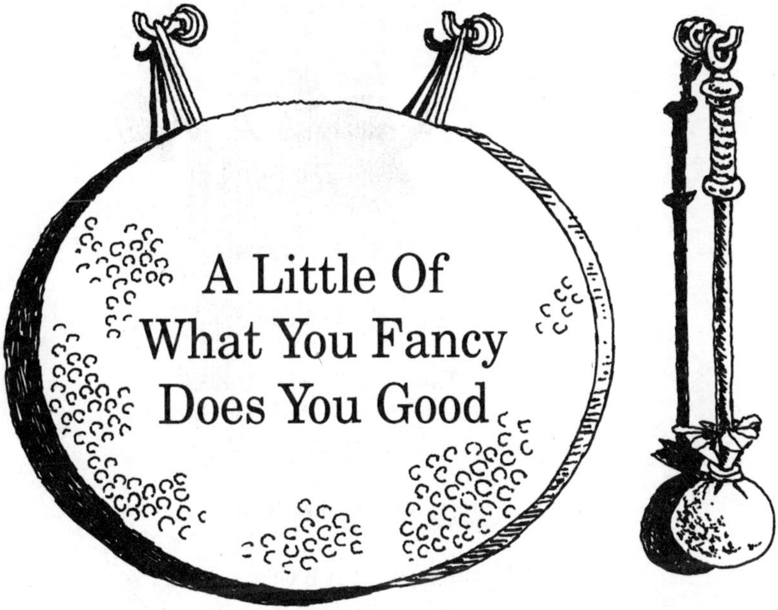

YOUR HEALTH IN LATER LIFE

by
Dr H B Gibson

Designed and illustrated by Rufus Segar

Third Age Press

London 1997

Third Age Press

ISBN 1 898576 09 2

First edition

Third Age Press Ltd, 1997
Third Age Press, 6 Parkside Gardens
London, SW19 5EY

Editor Dianne Norton

Designed, drawn and put into pages at the
MacSegar Press, Sandacre, Sandling
Hythe CT21 4HG

Printed and bound in Great Britain
by
Bell & Bain Limited
Glasgow

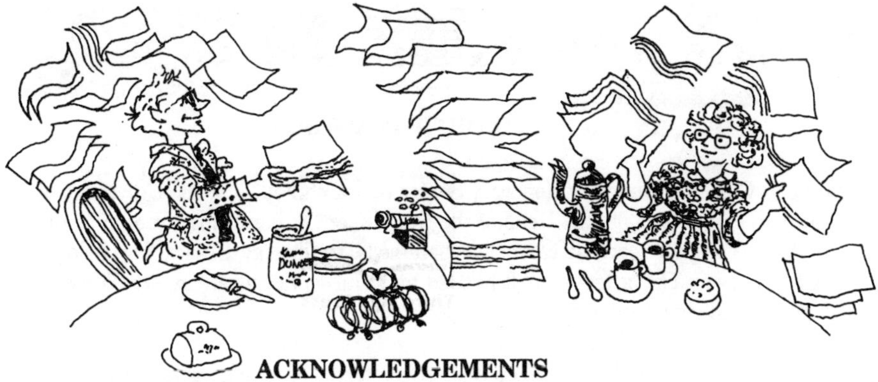

ACKNOWLEDGEMENTS

In this book I have chiefly followed the Reports on the health of older people that have been published as part of the Carnegie Inquiry Into the Third Age by Dr J Grimley Evans and his colleagues, and it is to them that I am chiefly indebted for their recent research findings and their practical recommendations. The interpretations that I have put upon their publications are, of course, my own. I am also greatly indebted to a number of other specialists in the health of the elderly who are too numerous to mention. I have tried to express these findings and recommendations in plain English and to avoid medical and other scientific jargon where possible, or at least to explain the terms used.

I have been very fortunate in that drafts of much of the book have been read by various medical specialists in different aspects of the health of older people and I have benefited greatly from their advice. I am particularly indebted to Dr John Benson, Dr Gordon Campbell, Dr Nicholas Coni, Dr Thomas Dening, Dr Duncan Forsyth, and Professor Kay-Tee Khaw for their help and encouragement.

In writing a book of this kind for the general public one aims not only to present sometimes controversial viewpoints about health in terms that are comprehensible to all, but to give the public 'a good read'. Here I am particularly indebted to Carol Graham who has read and advised on the whole manuscript, contributing her own ideas on health and its enjoyment, reining back some of my more exuberant hobby-horses and insisting always that I express myself in good English. The book has gained much from our many discussions of the chapters as they were written.

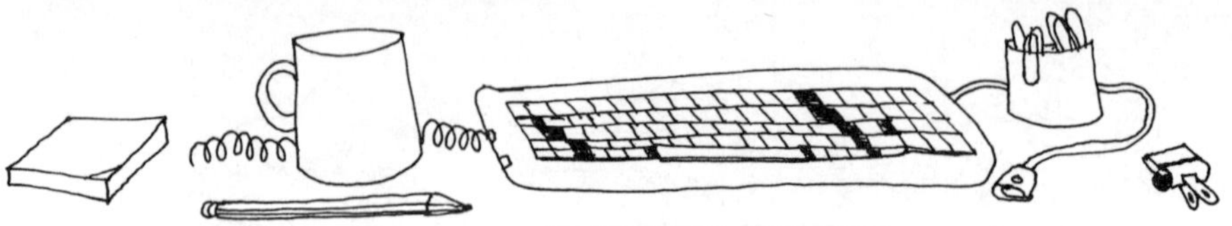

ABOUT THE AUTHOR

Dr H B Gibson is currently Honorary Senior Research Fellow at the University of Hertfordshire where he was Head of the Department of Psychology from 1970 to 1976. His 50-year teaching career has spanned Criminology, Clinical Psychology and Hypnosis. The latter interest has led him into service as an Expert Witness in criminal and civil court cases.

For the past 10 years he has taken an active interest in matters gerontological. He is a tutor and active member of the University of the Third Age in Cambridge and lectures and writes on a broad sweep of Third Age issues.

He has written prolifically over the years on a wide range of topics including contributions to journals of a humanist, sceptical and anarchist orientation. Notable publications include:

Love in Later Life London: Peter Owen Ltd 1997

On the Tip of Your Tongue: Your Memory in Later Life
London: Third Age Press 1995

Psychology, Pain and Anaesthesia H B Gibson (Ed)
London: Chapman Hall 1993

Emotional and Sexual Adjustment in Later Life. In *Ageing, Independence and the Life Course* (Eds. S Arber & M Evandrou)
London: Jessica Kingsley Publications 1993

Love, Sex and Power in Later Life London: Freedom Press 1992

The Emotional and Sexual Lives of Older People: A Manual for Professionals
London: Chapman & Hall 1991

The Nature of Hypnosis In E Karas (Ed)
Current Issues in Clinical Psychology New York: Plenum Publishing Co. 1987

Pain and its Conquest London: Peter Owen Ltd 1982

Hans Eysenck: The Man and His Work London: Peter Owen Ltd 1981

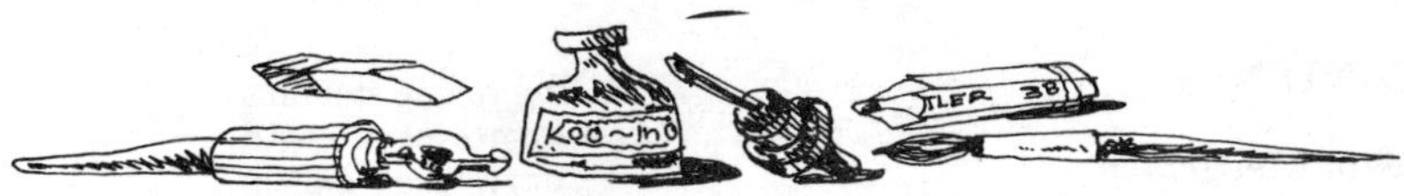

ABOUT THE ILLUSTRATOR

Rufus Segar is a designer as well as an illustrator. For 30 years under *The Economist* umbrella he worked away at devising charts, maps and pictorial diagrams to support economic texts; these were mainly written by researchers of *The Economist Intelligence Unit*. For most of that time he was freelance, he had learnt the trade by watching others while employed by manufacturers, agencies and publishers in his 20s.

The arrival of Apple Macintoshes in 1984 gradually made typography and chart making witless and ubiquitous. Realising that computers could not draw or write he left London for Hythe six years ago and turned himself into a topographer and desk top publisher. Books to look for:

Cockney Alphabet R Segar London: Max Parrish 1964
A LOST MASTERPIECE OF DESIGNED CARTOGRAPHIC DIAGRAMS:
The Atlas of Europe (Eds. R C Croucher & M C MacDonald)
Edinburgh & London: J Bartholomew and F Warne 1974

Publications still in print and easily got:
COMIC ILLUSTRATIONS FOR SERIOUS BOOKS:
In *The Economist* Pocket Books series:
The Economist Pocket Style Book 1986
Pocket Lawyer S Berwin 1987
Pocket Taxpayer B Sabine 1987
Pocket Guide to Business Taxes B Sabine 1988
On the Tip of Your Tongue: Your Memory in Later Life Dr H B Gibson
London: Third Age Press 1995
Flood, Fire, and Sudden Death in Old Hythe D Rayner
Hythe, Kent: Hythe Civic Society 1996
Spicer's Seventy Years S&L Spicer Lympne, Kent: Spicer's of Hythe 1996

SERIOUS TOPGRAPHIC DRAWINGS OF KENT BUILDINGS WITH PEOPLE USING THEM:
Remember Hythe: The High Street 1902 – 1992
Hythe, Kent: The MacSegar Press 1992 (a trove and still in print)
To support the fabric: all in print, £1 apiece, send for a set to keep the rain out:
Remember St Martin's Cheriton, Folkestone 1993
Remember St Peter & St Paul Saltwood, Hythe (3 parts) 1993 & 1994
Remember The Watermill at Hythe Hythe: Imperial Hotel 1994
For Hythe Civic Society:
The Town Hall of Hythe, One of the Cinque Ports D Rayner 1994
Our Time in Hythe: Review 1945 – 1995 G Roberts (Ed) 1995

CONTENTS

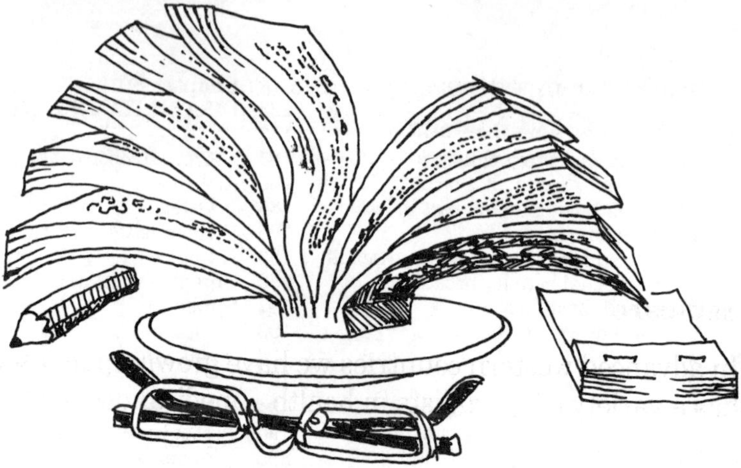

INTRODUCTION

This book is about the achievement and maintenance of health in later life, a period which is roughly defined as the years after retirement from full-time employment and family responsibility, and which has now come to be called the Third Age. I have based the book broadly on the findings and recommendations regarding health of Dr John Grimley Evans and his colleagues working on the Carnegie Third Age Inquiry. Their extensive *Report* ends with the words:

> The Third Age is not a short rest before dependency or death. It is an important and lengthening stage of the life cycle which nearly all of us will experience. With thought and preparation it can be made vastly more rewarding.

The main title of the book, which refers to the saying 'A little of what you fancy does you good', is my own idea, and throughout the chapters I seek to explain and justify it in the light of the most modern research findings of scientists of all branches of health-care which are conveyed here impartially in simple language. That many people do not look after their health as well as they might is partly due to lack of information, and partly to a conviction which is embodied in the pessimistic adage, 'All the best things in life are either illegal, immoral or fattening'. I hope to convince you of the falsity of this adage, and in fact to reconcile Dionysus, the god of wine and rejoicing with Asclepius, the god of health.

Self-care

In advanced western countries we have grown up in a society that has a variety of specialists in health – medical doctors, nurses, dentists, health-visitors etc. – and this has had the unfortunate effect of inducing in many people an attitude of passivity towards their own health. There is a tendency to think that it is 'their' business to keep 'us' healthy, whereas we should realize that health is our own responsibility.

To some degree this opinion was fostered in the past by many doctors who adopted a posture of extreme paternalism towards their patients: 'Just take the medicine I've prescribed for you Mrs Smith, and you'll be all right. Come and see me again in a month's time. Next patient please.' Such a doctor might confide to colleagues, 'God knows what's wrong with the old biddy – what does she expect at the age of 70? I've given her *x y z* which should do her no harm, and I expect she'll last for a bit longer.'

Such doctors strongly discouraged their patients from asking questions, implying that such was the ignorance of lay people that they could not begin to understand the mysteries of medicine and of their own bodies. They were simply to do as they were told, and to trust the doctor to know best in all things. Happily, this medical attitude has largely, but not entirely, passed away, and more modern doctors now encourage their patients to try to understand the working of their own bodies and the principles of healthy living.

The waiting-room of the doctors' practice I attend has a large library of books and pamphlets which patients are welcome to borrow. Such publications explain in simple language what is known about many common conditions from A (arthritis, allergies, asthma . . . to Z (zoster – the herpes virus that gives us shingles). They deal with the principles of health and how to cope with the various disorders which we may all suffer from occasionally.

Good modern doctors no longer fear to admit their ignorance. You are less likely to be fobbed of with some Graeco-Latin word (which merely means a sore stomach) and a bottle of pills when a doctor has no idea what's up with you. This great increase in honesty between doctor and patient is partly due to the fact that nowadays there are many really effective drugs and treatments, which have replaced the placebos and dummy treatments that used to be all too common. With modern medical methods the various possible causes of your disorder will be investigated, and if nothing is found you will be told this. Medical science is still expanding, and this applies especially with regard to the health of people in later life.

Due to the great advances that have been made in healthy living during this century we have the gift of about 20 to 30 extra years of life, and much of it will be spent in what is now known as the Third Age after our full-time working lives are over. This has never happened before in the history of the world, and so it is understandable that there is still much to be learnt about health in later life.

Specialists in what used to be called 'Geriatric Medicine' and is now called 'Medical Care of the Elderly' (so as not to hurt the feelings of older people like you and me) can be excused when they have to admit quite frankly that they cannot cure or explain all the aches or pains of their patients.

Medicine has learnt a great deal over a long period of time by the empirical study of people in sickness and in health, but such patients have been overwhelmingly the young and middle-aged, because there weren't so many oldies around in the past. Now doctors are confronted with ever-growing numbers of older patients who don't always react in the same way as those who are younger, or have the same problems. You must not expect doctors to deliver perfect health or miracles.

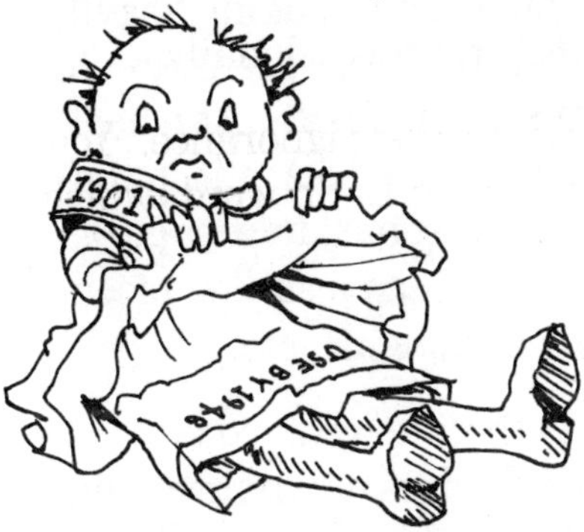

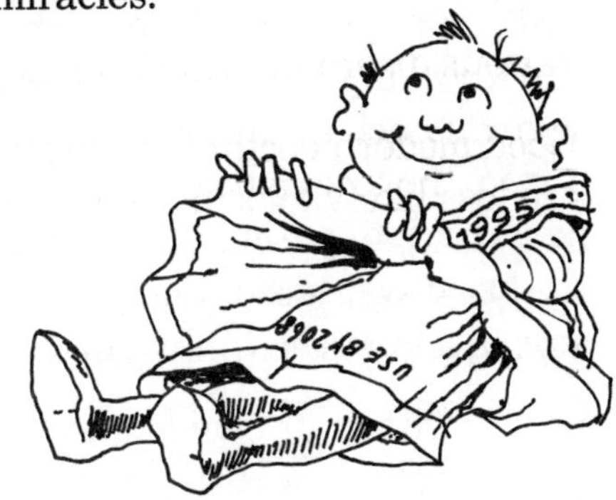

We should not under-rate the enormous benefits that orthodox medicine has conferred on us; the general improvement in health has been one of the greatest success stories of the present century. In 1901 the life expectancy at birth for males was 45 years. Now in the 1990s it is 73 years. For women it is even slightly better – from 49 years at birth to 79 years. This gain of approximately 30 years added to the life-span has largely been due to improvements in public health, the population becoming better educated and able to take advantage of the great strides that medicine and allied sciences have made in conquering disease and promoting positive health by advising on hygiene, better diet and housing.

It should be noted that public health measures – better housing, sanitation, control of factory conditions etc. – have made more impact on the population than the curative medicine that is practised in surgeries, clinics and hospitals. The incidence of tuberculosis, which used to be a common scourge in the population, was already waning in the 1940s before the introduction of drugs that were effective in its treatment.

In later life you can't do much about errors of the past that have affected your health, but one cheering finding in the researches of the Carnegie Third Age Inquiry is that in many aspects of health it is never too late to benefit from giving up deleterious habits with which you used to punish your body, such as smoking heavily and knocking back too much of the hard stuff. If you are trying to keep an ancient car running on the road you shouldn't just wheel it into the local garage every time it conks out and leave it to the mechanics to put it right. You should acquire some knowledge of the basic systems of the machine, even if you need a skilled mechanic to adjust the timing, de-coke the ancient engine, etc.

So it is with your own health. Your GP is there to give expert advice and, if necessary, to de-coke your cylinders or whatever, but your doctor cannot live your daily life for you. It is up to you to take responsibility for your health. No one would suggest that you should study medical textbooks, try to diagnose complex diseases, or try to dose yourself with powerful drugs, but you should take control of those matters that are within your province.

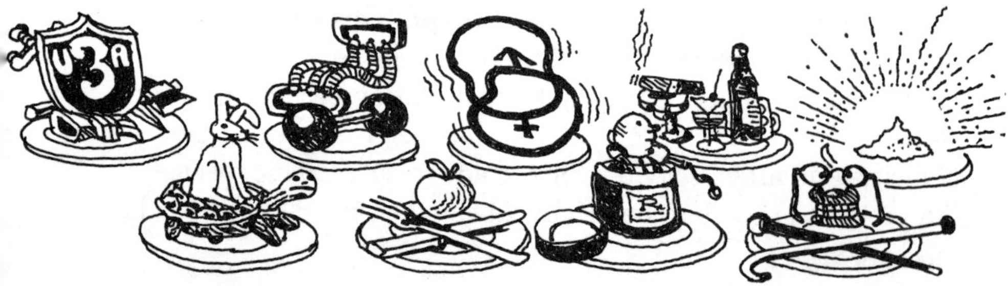

The Chapters

In Chapter 1 the nature of the Third Age and the challenges it presents to our health and daily living is addressed. First it is necessary to define what we mean by 'health', a term that is used in different ways by different people. I define health in terms of enjoying yourself with every prospect of continuing to do so with a life-style that does not threaten you with untimely disability and dependence. Certain basic needs are necessary for the fulfilment of a healthy and vigorous life, and prominent among them are the need for autonomy and the ability come to terms with a changing society. A number of social issues are discussed in this chapter which do not concern your relations with doctors and other health-care workers directly, but are nevertheless essential for healthy living, such as the need for a home which is not just a place to stay but a place where you feel in control of the environment.

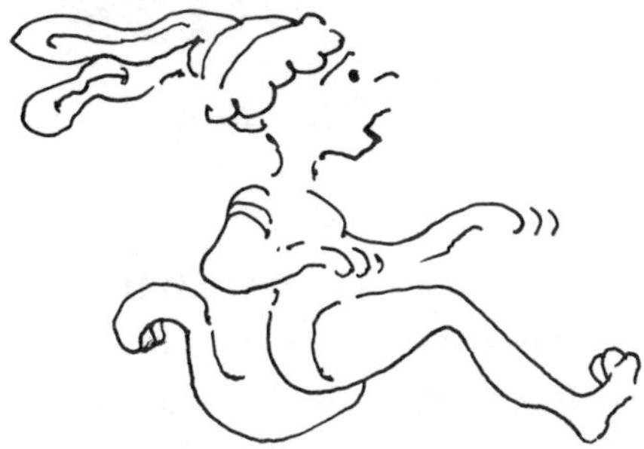

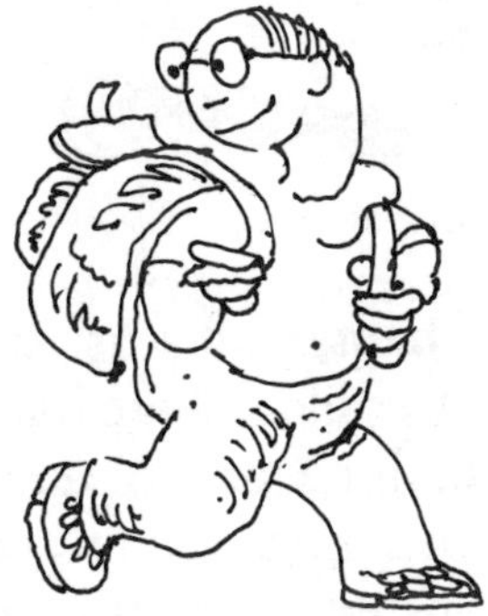

As we get older we become more unalike each other in a number of important ways: for instance, we age at very different rates as regards our physical fitness, and how we react to the surroundings in which we live.

Chapter 2 lists a number of ways in which older people differ from one another, and discusses the implications of these differences. Contemporary society tends to emphasize the fact that everyone has equal rights, and to combat unfair discrimination: this is certainly to be encouraged in a democracy, but it may be confused with a claim that we are all equal and to overlook important individual differences. People are not all the same because they are 'old': superficially they may appear to be an identifiable group because they tend to have grey hair, wrinkles and a pension, but the stereotype of 'the elderly', which is embodied in literature, tradition and much popular humour, can be very misleading. This chapter suggests that you should insist upon your right to be an individual with capacities, wishes, interests, and needs that have nothing to do with your chronological age.

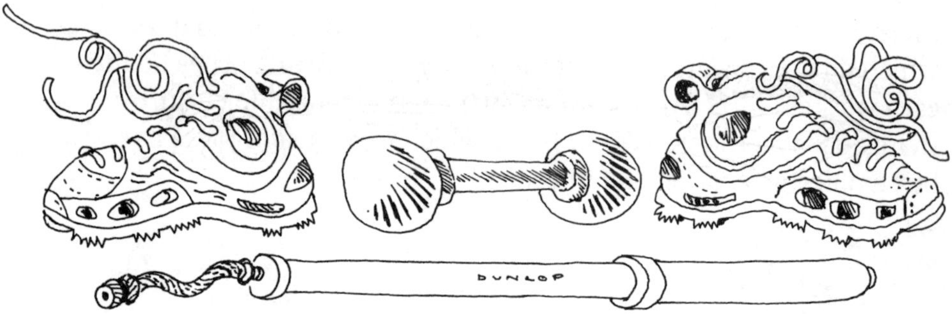

Chapter 3 discusses how much physical exercise should be taken in later life. There has been considerable research into this matter, and the most recent findings show that, on average, the amount of exercise taken by people in the Third Age is simply not enough to ensure their optimum health. There are several reasons that account for this, some of them resulting from a number of false beliefs about exercise which can be characterized as 'old wives' tales'. The misconceptions that lead people to become 'couch potatoes' are described and examined in detail.

It is admitted that physical fitness does inevitably decline with age, even without any pathological conditions being present, but our object should be to minimize this decline as much as possible. The concept of the 'fitness gap' is discussed – that is, the gap between the level of average fitness at any age that is easily attainable and the more often found lower level which is due to deleterious habits and not taking enough exercise. Advice is given about regaining and maintaining fitness in later life without attempting to adopt an unpleasantly spartan regime.

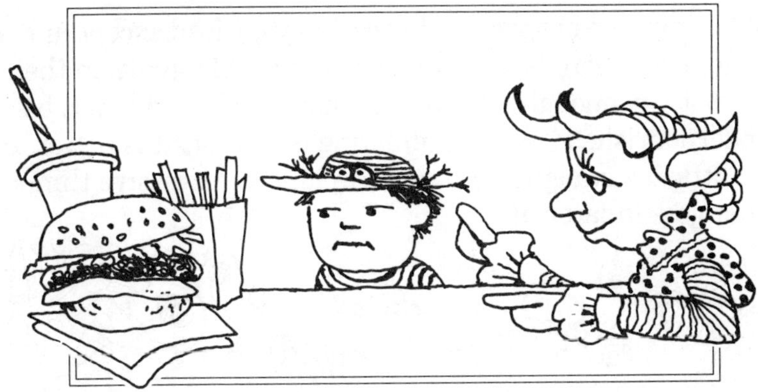

The saying 'A little of what you fancy does you good' in relation to diet is examined in Chapter 4, and is, on the whole, upheld. Any discussion of diet has to contend with arguments that are advanced on political and ethical grounds which are not necessarily valid.

It is not my purpose to take sides on issues such as vegetarianism; I simply want to explain what is known about food and its relation to health, and to quote the opinions of eminent dieticians who base their advice on scientific research. Food has always been the subject of some quite eccentric faddists, and a few of their diets are described and examined. Unfortunately, there is a lot of money to be made by promoting the sale of some so-called 'health' foods and food additives about which totally unjustifiable claims are made.

In more recent years elderly people have become specially targeted as a group who may be profitably exploited by claiming that the common disabilities of later life such as rheumatism can be cured by certain allegedly miraculous foods and additives which are very highly priced but of no real value.

The general recommendation given in Chapter 4 is that to maintain health you should have a good mixed diet and that there is no need for any sort of special additives to your food except under medical advice. There is some danger that people living on their own may not pay enough attention to their meals and hence become undernourished. While overeating is unwise, it is better to be just a little overweight than underweight for excessive thinness has its dangers in later life.

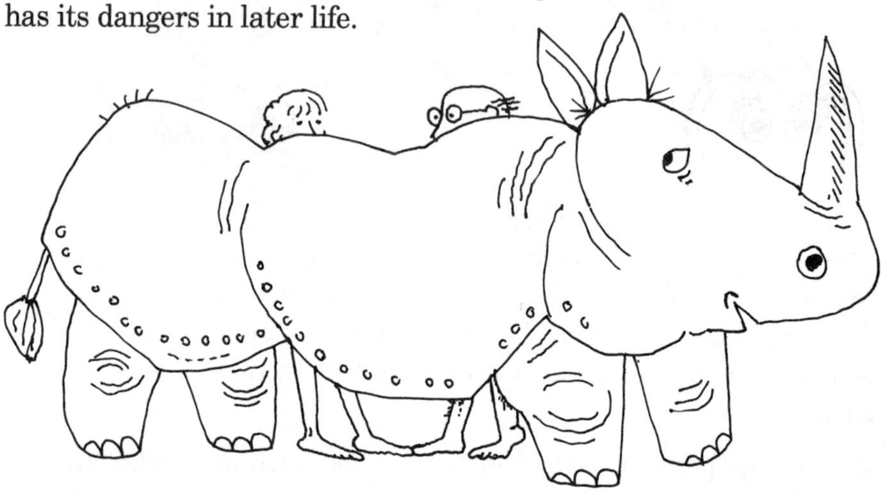

Chapter 5 deals with the sex-lives of older people. While some people may be perfectly healthy and happy with no sexual activity, it is more usual for men and women to want some form of sexual fulfilment whatever their age. Great changes in public attitudes to and knowledge about sexuality have occurred in the latter part of this century.

In the famous Kinsey researches into human sexuality in the 1940s and 1950s, they did not trouble to interview many older people because it was assumed that after a certain age they had no interest at all in sex. Since then it has become generally recognized that there is no cessation of such interest with ageing, both in the emotional and physical spheres. Obviously as bodily vigour declines, physical activity becomes less important, but men and women still fall in love at quite advanced ages, and may form new relationships of a stable and rewarding nature.

A large part of this chapter is devoted to countering the considerable amount of false information about sexual matters that is still current as a legacy from the Victorian era. Many doctors who were quite sensible in other matters used to retail an extraordinary body of nonsense about the relationship between sexuality and health, and it is important to dispel these myths.

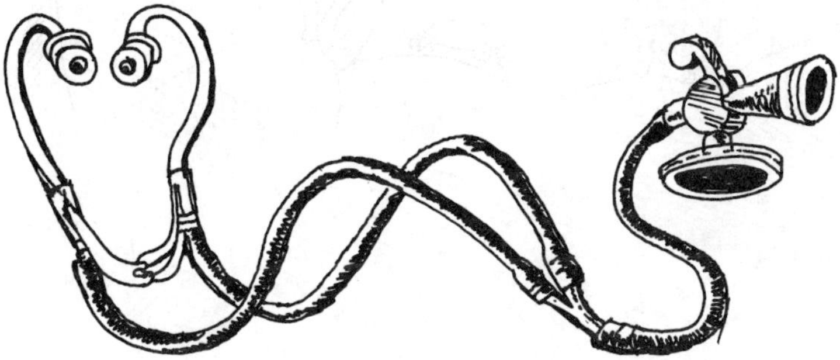

The relations between doctors and patients are explored in some detail in Chapter 6. As mentioned previously, the medical world has undergone some significant changes in the last half-century, and doctors have become far less authoritarian with their patients.

Older patients who have grown up to expect their doctors to be all-knowing in health matters (or pretending to be so) have had to re-adjust to a situation where the primary responsibility for their health lies in their own hands, medical and other health services being available to them more in a specialist advisory capacity.

Strangely enough, these changes have resulted in a great growth in all kinds of 'alternative therapy', much of which is anti-scientific in orientation, and because it is outside the National Health Service, can be immensely profitable for the practitioners who do not necessarily have any professional training or standards of ethical control. Some details of the attempts that have been made by the British Medical Association to come to terms with 'alternative therapy' are given in this chapter.

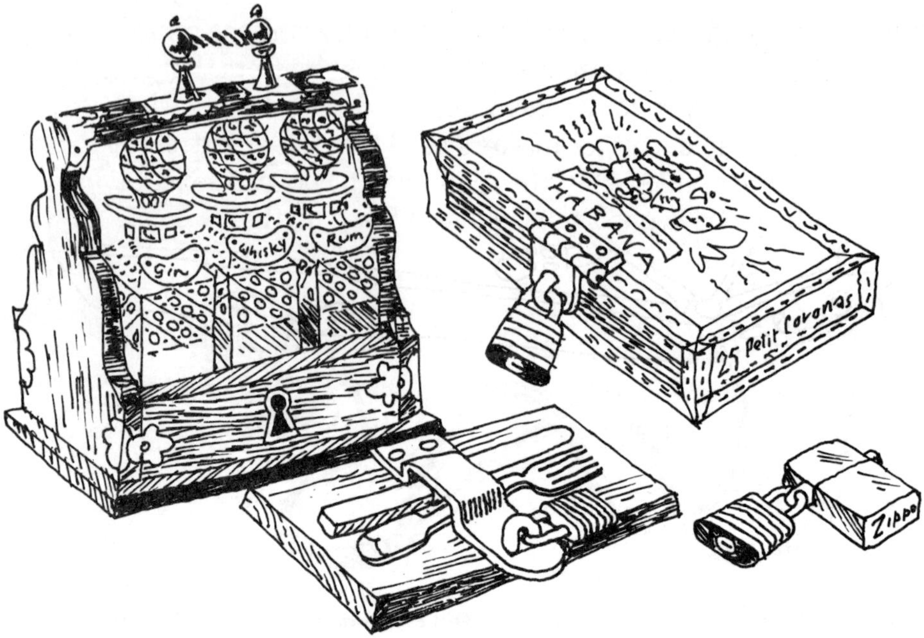

Chapter 7 deals with 'The pitfalls of later life', that is the hazards that are attached to pleasures such as eating, drinking alcohol, and smoking, especially in the latter part of our lives. It is now generally known that serious and life-threatening diseases may result from over-indulgence in these pleasures, but if one is to maintain that 'A little of what you fancy does you good' the question arises how much is 'a little' and just what is the nature of the risks involved.

It is necessary to examine these matters in some detail, for we need to balance our pleasure and enhancement of the quality of life against the possible consequences of over-indulgence.

As heart-attacks, cancer and strokes are major causes of disability and death in later life, these three diseases are discussed, and some interesting although highly speculative research is described in the course of examining the relationship of our habits and general way of life to breakdown in health.

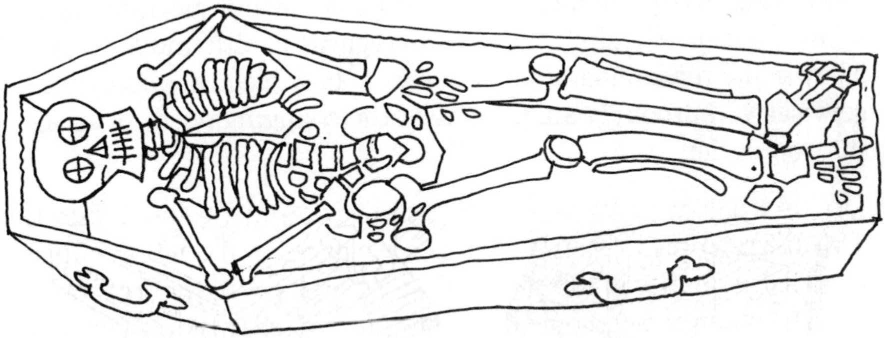

This book is about health and its maintenance, but it would be hardly realistic if the major causes of ill-health in the later years of life were not identified and possible ways of avoiding and mitigating them discussed. This is done in Chapter 8 where it is pointed out that in most cases there are some active remedial steps that can be taken in later life, but to some extent factors in childhood or even in our pre-natal condition have pre-determined later weaknesses.

It is also a truism that one of the best ways of securing a long and healthy life is to pick our parents carefully – i.e. what happens to us in life is partly due to our inherited genetic programming. We have to learn what is the best we can do within the constraints our individual nature imposes on us.

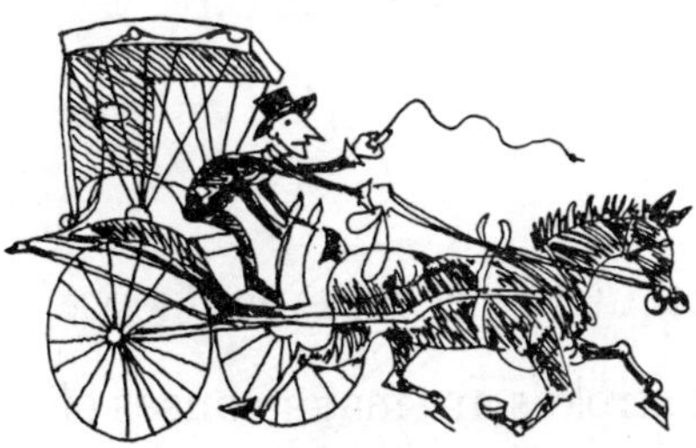

The title of Chapter 9 – *The One-hoss Shay* – is taken from a poem by Oliver Wendell Holmes that has formed the inspiration of a number of influential scientists to theorize about the future. They discuss the nature of mankind – our life-span, our mortality and what the future is likely to bring as regards health and longevity. They make reasonable predictions as to how medical and social services will probably adapt to meet the changing needs of an ageing population.

On the whole we have every reason to be optimistic and to face the Third Age with confidence, that is if we agree that what is important is the quality of life rather than its actual length. In times gone by when most people died very much earlier than their natural life-span – tragically so in the case of children – the major emphasis was on length of life, and some even speculated that we might even aspire towards immortality. Such idle dreams have been abandoned, and in this modern age reasonable people accept that we are mortal, and must make the best of the life that we have.

It is the optimism of the specialists in health-care that has made me choose the title for this book – *A little of what you fancy does you good* – and when you have read it, and understood it, I hope you will agree that it is a reasonable conclusion, and that it is the policy to adopt when looking after your health.

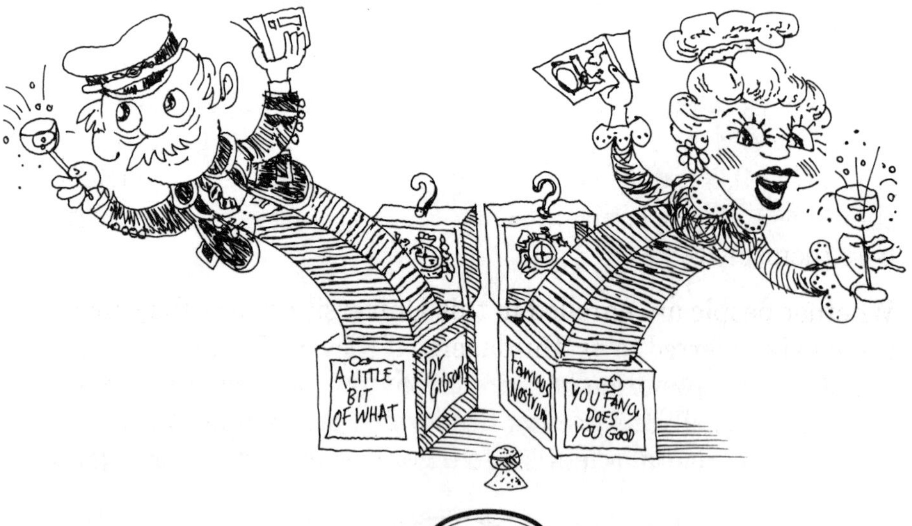

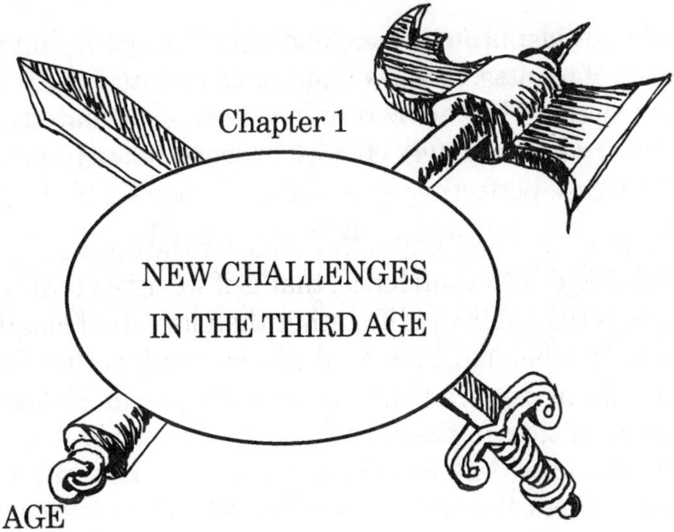

Chapter 1

NEW CHALLENGES IN THE THIRD AGE

THE THIRD AGE

The term the Third Age has come into general use largely through the writings of the eminent demographer and social historian Peter Laslett, who discussed the concept at length in his book *A Fresh Map of Life*. In France, Les Universités des Troisième Age were instituted in the 1970s when universities began to cater for the educational needs of people who were mainly past the age of retirement from paid full-time work, and wished to study all manner of subjects and to broaden their horizons generally.

Laslett, together with some colleagues, founded the first British University of the Third Age in 1981, and the movement has spread across the country, there now being over 300 local U3As with over 50,000 members. The general idea is that these U3As should be self-supporting and that study groups are led by members themselves.

Whether people are enrolled in this University or not, they have come to be referred to as 'thirdagers' if they conform to certain criteria: they are normally retired from full-time paid work, are relatively free of family responsibility and are in a position to occupy their leisure in fulfilling themselves in all manner of ways, just as students do in their undergraduate days, but not with the object of passing exams, obtaining qualifications and building a new career. They are certainly not closely bound to academic pursuits; if a thirdager chooses to spend his or her time visiting cathedrals, perfecting skill on the harmonica, birdwatching, building boats, or learning Chinese cooking, all these activities would come within the ambit of the University of the Third Age. However, it is not my purpose to describe the latter institution, but the concept of the Third Age.

The idea of mankind having several 'Ages', in the sense of separate periods of time in the life-course, is very ancient, and the number of these 'Ages' has varied greatly between different writers and philosophers. You may be familiar with the 'seven ages of Man' as they are described in Shakespeare's *As You Like It*. It makes sense to consider childhood and adolescence as a definite period during which the individual is dependent both economically and in terms of citizenship because he or she is being educated and acquiring skills wherewith to join the ranks of the productive working society.

Obviously we should refer to this period as the First Age. It does not do to be too precise as to actual chronicle markers: someone may have completed his apprenticeship while he is still a teenager and may already be a husband and father working at a full-time job. He has certainly progressed beyond his First Age. By contrast, another person who is many years past the 20th birthday and is still a full-time student should properly be classed as being within the First Age, although possessing all the political rights of citizenship.

The Second Age covers everyone who is part of the full-time working population (although they may sometimes be unemployed) and is normally engaged in such important matters as raising a family, building a career, and taking part in the social and political life of the community. It is a time that often involves some struggle, for if you have to earn a living at whatever job you can find, it may not be the ideal occupation for you, and you have to forgo the interests you would like to pursue, and postpone, except on a very part-time basis, any further education and self-improvement that you would dearly wish to acquire.

It is not just that in the Second Age you have to work to earn your own living: much of your energy may have to go to contributing to the support of those who are in the First Age (your own children, if any, and other people's children at school) and indeed all those – the sick, the unemployed, the infirm – who are in any way dependent on the public purse – which is supplied by the taxes you pay. In a sense too, you have to work to support someone who does not yet exist – yourself in old age. Whether you do this by the old method of hoarding gold in a sock, or by the modern method of paying into a pension fund, it comes to much the same thing.

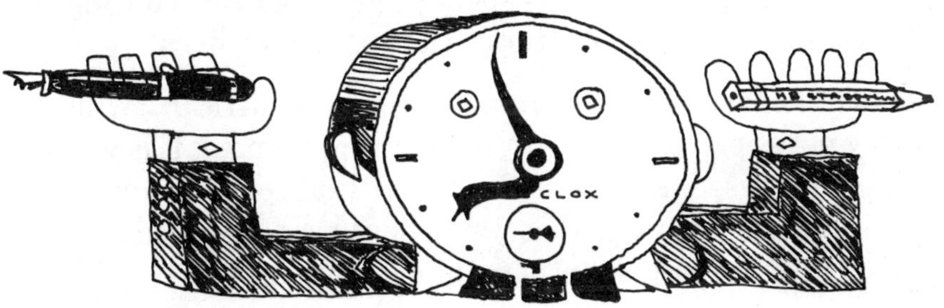

The Third Age, as conceived by contemporary writers, is a very modern concept, and has not really existed in history until the latter half of the twentieth century. This new phenomenon is the outcome of two things: first, the practice of family limitation which began among the middle-class about 1870, and second, the greatly increased health and longevity of the population that has been occurring during the present century due to advances in public health (improved sanitation, diet, better housing, clean water etc.), and the effective control and prevention of infectious diseases.

When the birth-rate drops the effect on the population structure is not manifest for about half a century, but it inevitably means that the proportion of older people in the community will increase relative to the proportion who are young. In the 1870s the proportion of people over the age of 60 in the population was only about 5%; this rose to about 10% by the 1920s, and by the 1990s it was over 15%. However, two things were significant about the small populations of elderly people at the earlier dates: they could not be expected to go on living for so very long, and they were not as healthy and robust as elderly people are today.

Thus, for the first time in history there is now a relatively large body of people who have completed their period of full-time work, career building and family responsibility, are quite active and robust, and who can confidently look forward to another 20 or 30 years of uninterrupted leisure to spend as they please, within the constraints of their economic circumstances. This is the period of the Third Age, and this book is about preserving health during this age, and using it to live constructive and satisfying lives.

I was told the following humorous story by an American. While you may not appreciate this sort of American humour, it is worth repeating because it expresses the new attitude of people entering the Third Age, an attitude that would have been regarded as quite reprehensible by most of our parents' generation:

> There was a Roman Catholic priest, an American lawyer and a Rabbi in conversation, and they began to debate the question of when life really begins. The priest gave it as his judgement that life begins at the moment of conception and is sacred ever after; the lawyer said that the matter was very complex but he would agree with whatever the Supreme Court decreed; the Rabbi said, 'Look, you guys have got it all wrong; of course life really begins when the kids leave home and the dog dies.

This may represent contemporary Third Age attitude in America, but when holidaying in Devon last year I was able to buy a car-sticker which reads:

> **RETIRED AND HAPPY**
>
> SPENDING OUR KIDS' INHERITANCE

IS THERE A FOURTH AGE?

It has been proposed that we should consider in our scheme a final and Fourth Age, characterized by dependency and decrepitude, which is, of course, referred to as the 'seventh age of Man' in Shakespeare's *As You Like It*:

Last scene of all

That ends this strange eventful history,

Is second childishness, and mere oblivion,

Sans eyes, sans teeth, sans taste, sans everything.

Although this concept has been accepted by many people, I do not think it is necessary. If I am in my Third Age and fall ill at Christmas and remain a dependent invalid until next midsummer when I die, presumably I am to be referred to as being in the Fourth Age for the intervening six months. This may have been a frequent occurrence before the days of effective medicine, but with the modern techniques that are available, I may not die at midsummer but be restored to health and vigour – have I then popped back into the Third Age to continue my active life?

Later in this book I will consider more than one case of elderly men and women who have apparently entered a period of swift decline towards death, but who have been restored to normal health by medical treatment.

My objection to the concept of the Fourth Age is that if it was ever a useful one it is now outmoded, and is a very pessimistic and demeaning label to give to anyone. If I fall ill and am hence dependent on those around me, how long must the period of dependence last before I am to be labelled as being in my Fourth Age? A month, six months, a year? Geriatricians are becoming more and more wary of diagnosing anyone as being in a 'terminal' condition, for as medical science continues to advance such a diagnosis becomes less certain, and there have been some remarkable recoveries in later life.

The concept of the Fourth Age was made use of in the eighteenth century by Swift in his *A Voyage to Laputa*, where he introduces a terrible satire on old age – the Struldbruggs. These people were condemned by nature never to die despite their miserable condition of suffering from all the infirmities of age, both physical and mental, to an ever-increasing extent, yet unable to be released from them by death.

The ideal that we aspire to in our society is to ensure that everyone is healthy and active until the day they die, and that there should be no period of life that resembles the Fourth Age. We all must die some day. and it is uncertain what the natural span of life is for human beings.

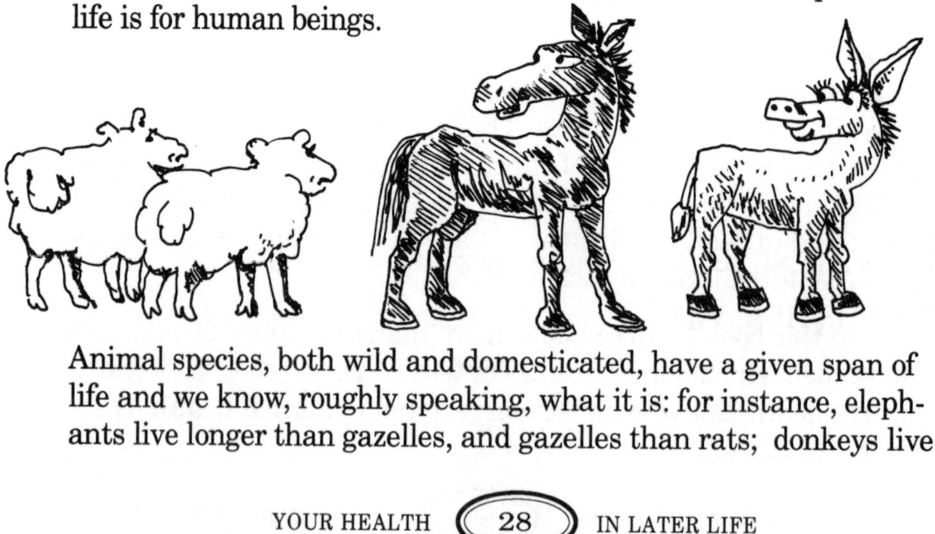

Animal species, both wild and domesticated, have a given span of life and we know, roughly speaking, what it is: for instance, elephants live longer than gazelles, and gazelles than rats; donkeys live longer than horses, and horses than sheep. Each species appears to be programmed to live for a certain span of time, give or take a few years, and presumably this applies to the human species as well. According to *The Bible:*

> *We spend our years as a tale that is told.*
>
> *The days of our years are threescore years and ten;*
>
> *And if by reason of strength they be fourscore years,*
>
> *Yet is their strength labour and sorrow;*
>
> *For it is soon cut off, and we fly away.*

It is of great interest that this Psalm is over 2,000 years old yet the span of life depicted there is not greatly different from that which we expect today, although now we would not agree that the added robustness of those who live to 80 years and longer is 'labour and sorrow'.

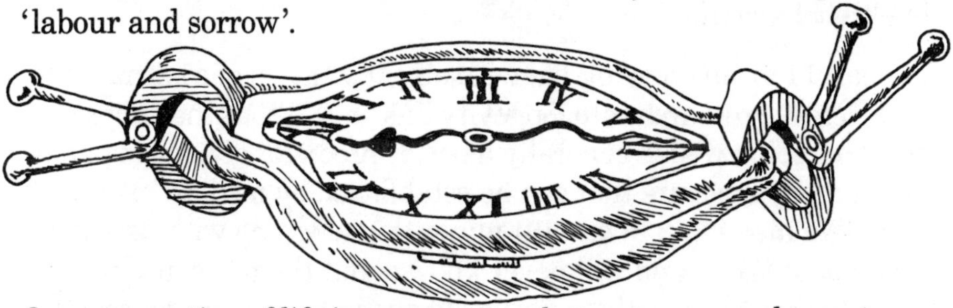

Our expectation of life is now greater, but not very much greater; we do not know what the 'natural' span of human life is, and what seems more important to most people is the quality of later life rather than its length. None of us would like to resemble the Struldbruggs that Swift invented in his satire, who continued to live on and on but were wracked by every sort of misery.

WHAT IS HEALTH?

Many people have defined health differently, and I want to make it clear that in this book I mean something positive by health, and not just absence of disease. Consider this definition which was given by two writers concerned with health-care:

> Health behaviour is any activity undertaken by a person believing himself to be healthy, for the purpose of preventing disease or detecting it in an asymptomatic state.

Is this what you mean by health behaviour? I hope not, because if so I will think that when you go out for a nice country walk among the fields you do not look around at the beauties of nature but keep your eyes firmly on the grass verges in case an adder pops out and bites you. What is described above seems to me to be a sort of super-alert hypochondria – 'Dare I drink a second glass of sherry or will it injure my brain? Dare I risk a sandwich at the buffet as it may be spread with saturated fat and therefore be a danger to my heart? Should I have carefully observed the cleanliness of the ice-cream vendor's hands, and should I throw this cornet away?' To my mind this is not 'health behaviour'.

By health I mean enjoying life with an expectation of continuing to do so. Scientific research into longevity has shown that the subjective feeling of being well is generally a better predictor of a long span of life than any measure that can be established by medical examination. We may have all sorts of minor things wrong with us and not know about them, and will never know about them because we may live happily and robustly to a ripe old age in happy ignorance of them.

When a very old person dies it is generally rather uncertain what is the cause of death. Something has to be put down on the death certificate, but it might well be several other things. To quote a very eminent geriatrician, Dr Grimley Evans:

> The reductionist tradition of seeking a unifying diagnosis for a patient's manifold symptoms and signs may mislead a doctor encountering an old person who may be more likely to be suffering from two or three common diseases than from one rare one. Interactions between multiple diseases and their treatments are a further source of difficulty in the practice of geriatric medicine.

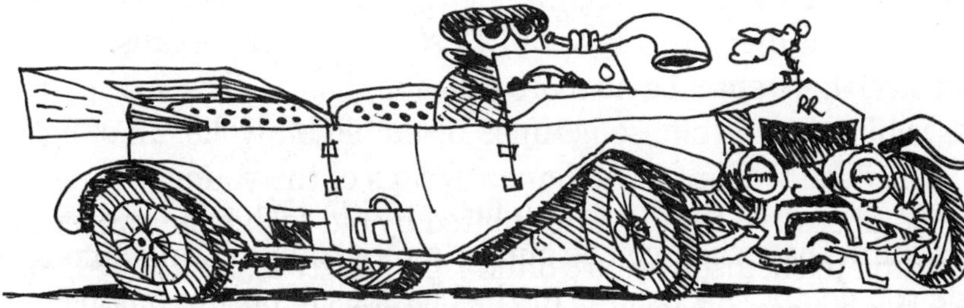

I certainly do not advocate neglecting any symptom of illness that you may notice; if you run a very old car and you hear a suspicious knock developing in the engine you take it round to the garage immediately, and thus save yourself expensive repairs later; so you should do the same with yourself when you have a sound reason to suspect that something is going wrong. Your car needs an annual MOT when it is over a statutory age.

When you are over a certain age (which is fixed quite arbitrarily at 75) you are entitled to an annual inspection. What a 'sound reason' is must be left to the good judgement of you and your doctor. In practice you will be told if you are worrying over trifles, but it is handy to know if you have blood-pressure normal for your age, no sign of diabetes, no suspicious lumps, a heart that sounds in passable condition, and similar health markers.

CAKES AND ALE

Some writers of books and journals about health, both scientific and popular, seem to have got paediatrics muddled with geriatrics, for when they are addressing, or writing about older people they seem to assume that when we have reached a certain age we have indeed entered a 'second childhood' and are to be addressed and discussed as though we are children dependent on Nanny to tell us what to do – what not to eat and drink, how not to behave, and all the most awful things that will probably happen to us if we do not heed their dire warnings. I am moved to respond, like Sir Toby Belch in Shakespeare's *Twelfth Night,* when he was reproved for his indulgent living by Malvolio, 'Dost thou think, because thou art virtuous, there shall be no more cakes and ale?' The young, in prescribing for the old, sometimes resemble Malvolio: an enlightened medical writer in *The Lancet* writes of the younger generation 'so liberal, so free, so uninhibited by old-fashioned conventions according to themselves, are often rigid, narrow, puritanical, and censorious when it comes to the behaviour of older citizens.'

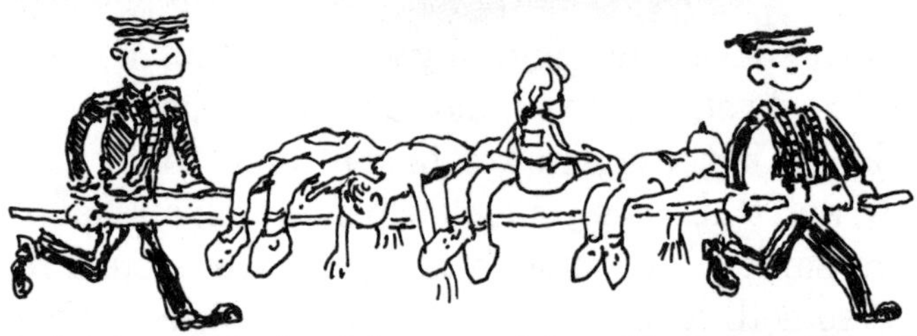

Some professionals in health-care of the elderly are like the St John's Ambulance Brigade at a marathon: they judge the success of the event in terms of the stragglers who drop out along the wayside with twisted ankles, blistered feet and strained hearts, and pay little attention to the majority who reach the finishing post, tired but successful.

In the marathon of life we aim to reach the end in that condition, a bit worn no doubt, but having had a happy and rewarding run right until the end. You cannot blame professional health-care workers for being rather overcautious, and sometimes talking like Nanny, for they cannot afford to take risks as you can. Most of the older people they see are not a normal sample of those in the Third Age who are healthy and independent, but a minority who are the sick and dependent, so it is quite natural that their view becomes somewhat biased.

When we reach the Third Age, many of us – perhaps most of us – will be a bit battered by our previous struggles, but even though you may now have a patch over one eye and a peg leg like Long John Silver, I insist that you can still be healthy, and aim to continue to be healthy, in terms of my definition of health which embraces enjoyment of life.

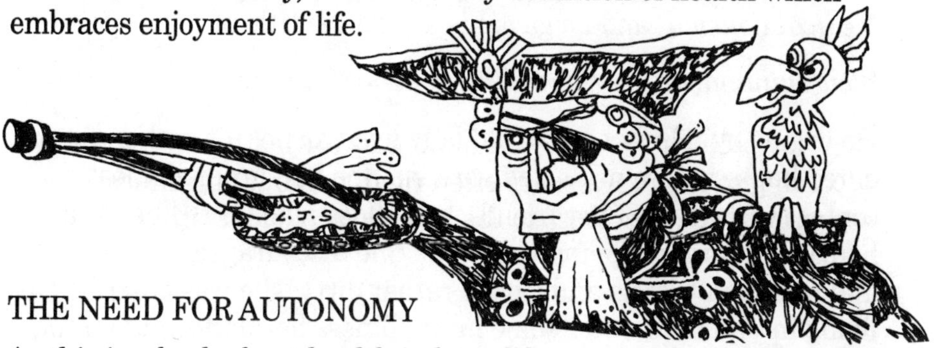

THE NEED FOR AUTONOMY

As this is a book about health in later life you may have expected it to start off with advice about diet, fresh air and exercise, and what medicines to take and not take. All these matters will be given attention in subsequent chapters, but what is just as important is your way of life and how you relate socially to the general community. It has been pointed out authoritatively that while about 25% of the troubles of later life are 'biogenic' (i.e. engendered by biological, etc, processes or forces) the remaining 75% are 'sociogenic'.

This means that quantitatively, the troubles that come through the ageing of your body, are in the minority compared to all the troubles that come through the way in which society treats its older people and relates to them, especially because of the circumstances of the rise of the new phenomenon of the Third Age which have been described above. Strangely enough, it was not a phenomenon which was anticipated and planned for.

One of the most important needs for the health of older people is autonomy, and to illustrate this I shall quote a quite extreme case. Contrary to popular opinion, very few retired people are so dependent that they have to live in residential accommodation of one kind or another – old people's homes and geriatric hospitals. It is reckoned that only about 3% of the retired population are in this category. You will note that I have written 'have to' but that is a matter of controversy among those responsible for social policy. My illustrative case was described by a doctor writing in the *British Medical Journal*, and he gave his article the title of :

Slow euthanasia or – She will be better off in hospital.

He begins by telling how an old lady lived alone in a rather dilapidated house with a neglected garden. She had gradually lost contact with most of her friends, and those who visited her and helped her with shopping were few. She discouraged home help and meals on wheels and looked rather dirty; she was described as living in 'squalor'. After some minor illness her doctor put strong pressure on her and persuaded her to go into hospital. The doctor reported:

> The patient is admitted, bathed, re-dressed, and within twenty-four hours may hardly be recognizable as the same person as the dirty, tattered old woman crouched at home by her fire. On the other hand the old woman crouched by her fire often had a good deal to say for herself, showed both individuality and determination, and could be self-assertive. In hospital, however, the same old woman may appear bewildered, restless, look around in perplexity and seem unable to express any need other than, perhaps, the desire to go home. At some point, perhaps after a fall, or because something in the patient's appearance causes concern, she is put to bed, within a day or two develops chest symptoms, and dies a day or two later.

This doctor goes on to say that in his hospital it was found that 25% of patients of this kind died within three weeks of admission, although some of them were physically healthy on admission.

I note that in this article the person in question is referred to at first as an 'old lady' when she is living independently, but when she has become a depersonalized patient in hospital she is called an 'old woman'. There is a subtle but significant difference between the two terms as commonly used. With the lessening of class distinctions among adults, the difference between 'ladies' and 'women' has become less important, but in later life they are reinstated, and there is a special meaning given to the term 'an old woman'.

This old lady's case, although extreme, illustrates the need for personal autonomy to make life worth living. Many people who are by no means poor, or living in squalor, exhibit the syndrome of giving up, losing their health, and just going into a decline when they lose their autonomy. There are now many, many women in later life who live alone, perhaps in houses rather too big for their present needs; fewer men are in this position, partly because there are many more women than men in the Third Age, and because men are more often living with a spouse in later life.

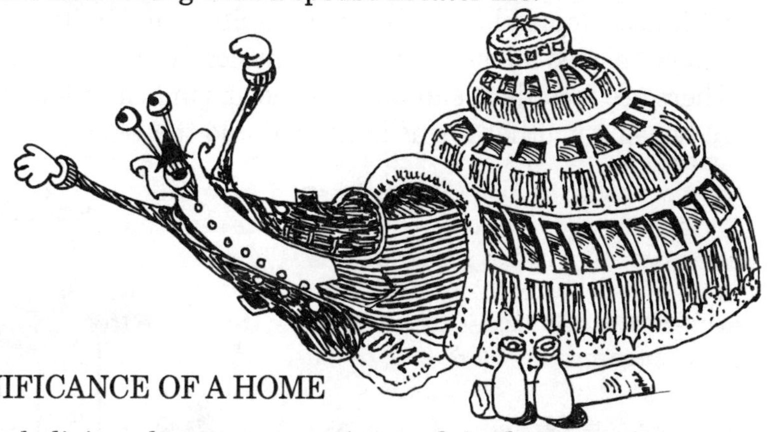

THE SIGNIFICANCE OF A HOME

Elderly people living alone are sometimes advised to move into another type of accommodation, perhaps in so-called 'sheltered housing', or to go to live with a middle-aged child or relative. If you are in this position you should be very cautious in taking such a decision; losing your accustomed home can be very traumatic indeed, far more so than you may realize. Your autonomy, your sense of living your individual, independent existence depends very much in later life on the home to which you are accustomed; without it you may feel like a snail deprived of its shell. There is a great deal of evidence to support this, and it may apply to communities as well as to individuals.

It was noted in the 1960s when a lot of the old neighbourhoods in London, sometimes designated rightly or wrongly as 'slums', were demolished, and the inhabitants moved into newly-built blocks of flats, the unexpected happened as far as the health of a lot of these re-housed people was concerned. The numbers attending the surgeries of the local doctors increased, patients complaining of all sorts of ill-defined disorders.

We are accustomed to thinking of public health partly depending on proper housing, and undoubtedly the worst types of housing were responsible for a variety of illnesses in earlier times, but most of the old property in the 1960s had at least minimal standards for decent living. The re-housing programme had deprived people of their accustomed homes and communities, and quite a number of people reacted adversely in their physical and mental health. There are records of similar breakdowns in health following re-housing in other towns in the UK and the USA.

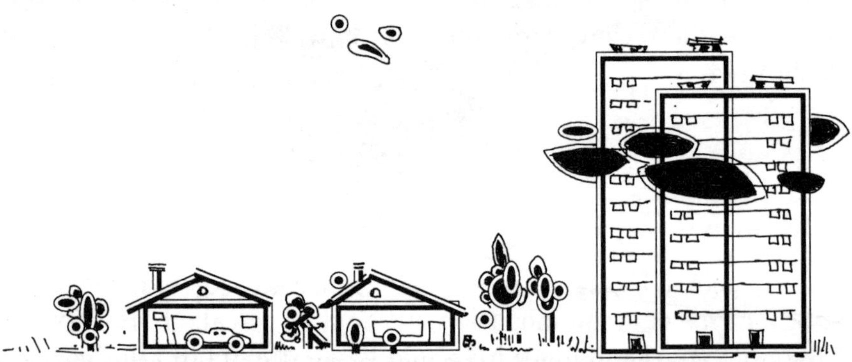

This phenomenon does not only apply to people losing their homes in working-class districts. A sad case is exemplified by what happened to a near neighbour of mine in a quite affluent middle-class neighbourhood. She was a widow living alone in a house that was too large for her needs. She was a very active lady who was very proud of her house and her tiny garden, both of which she kept in an immaculate condition. She had travelled widely, and her house was crammed with all sorts of relics of her travels, maintained beautifully, and she delighted to show visitors around to admire her home and its contents.

A sad family crisis necessitated the raising of a considerable sum of money, and she did this very unselfishly by selling her house and moving into a tiny flat. The flat was actually a newly-renovated alms-house that had been converted into quite an attractive little one-roomed dwelling, and her family thought that she would have less work to do without the house and garden that had taken up so much of her energies, and that now she could more enjoy her leisure in retirement.

This lady showed me her new flat, which was well-appointed, but of course all the excess furniture, bric-a-bac, and relics of her lifetime of travelling had been disposed of, and although she put a brave face on, and assured me how lucky she was to have such a place, she was plainly miserable. Not long after the move she had to go into hospital for an investigation, and when old friends went to see her there they were appalled to find that she had become withdrawn.

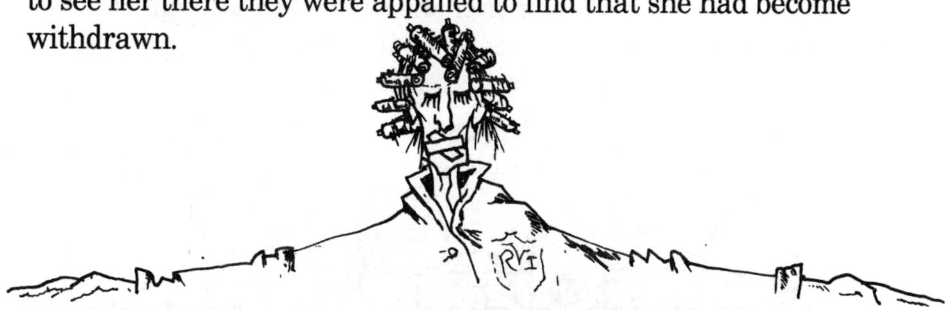

This brisk and proud lady, who was normally so talkative, seemed to have shrunk very rapidly into a pathetic 'old woman' who eventually refused to talk to anyone. As there appeared to be no medical reason for keeping her in the general hospital, and she had become utterly withdrawn and mute, she was moved to a psychiatric hospital where she soon died.

Many people who are rendered single in later life give up their accustomed homes and move in with their middle-aged children.

This is often successful and provides a satisfactory way of children providing care for their elderly parents when they need it. However, there are problems here that require very serious consideration. If you have stayed at the houses of your children or other relatives in the position of an honoured guest, year after year, such visits may have been delightful, but it may be quite another matter if you move in on a permanent basis, having given up your own home. After all, it is their home and not yours, and they have a right to run it as they see fit and not according to your standards.

When you were just a visitor you could perhaps laugh at the funny way they brought up the grandchildren, and perhaps twitted them when troubles ensued. But when a resident grandmother proves too strict and old-fashioned, or too foolishly indulgent, irritation may arise and she may be told to hold her tongue and not to interfere.

I need not enlarge on all the possible areas of unforeseen friction that may arise when a member of one generation attempts to live in the house of those of another when it is the younger generation who are in control and the older an interloper.

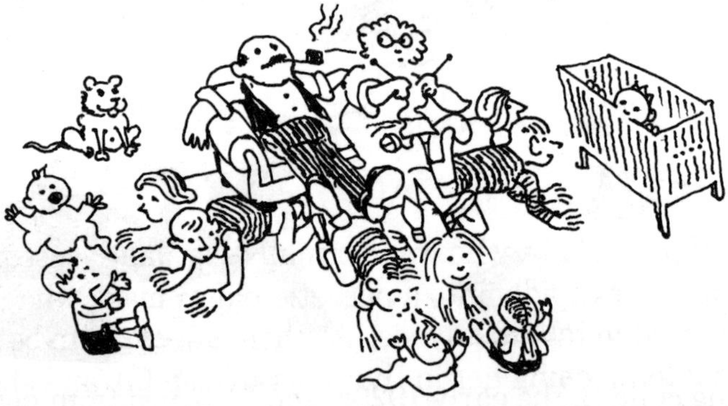

In the old days of the multigeneration family the older generation were in control of the household as patriarch or matriarch, but nowadays the position is generally reversed, and if the grandfather and grandmother figures have given up their own homes, and all the personal security and status that these homes meant to them, they are literally 'homeless' although living perhaps in a very comfortable house of another. It is, of course, impossible to say how many of these menages are successful, for what goes on is entirely private, and even if the arrangement proves to be a complete failure in terms of the happiness of those concerned, it is unlikely that grandad (who used to be such a dear old gentleman) will be turned out now he has become a nasty old curmudgeon, because he no longer has any home to go to.

COMING TO TERMS WITH THE NEW

One of the great challenges of later life that must be met involves coming to terms with a world that has changed. One of the unpleasant aspects of the stereotype of older people is that they are cantankerous, ill-tempered, complaining, censorious, prejudiced, and that they hate 'the young'. It is said that there is never smoke without fire, and so we should examine the causes of the fire.

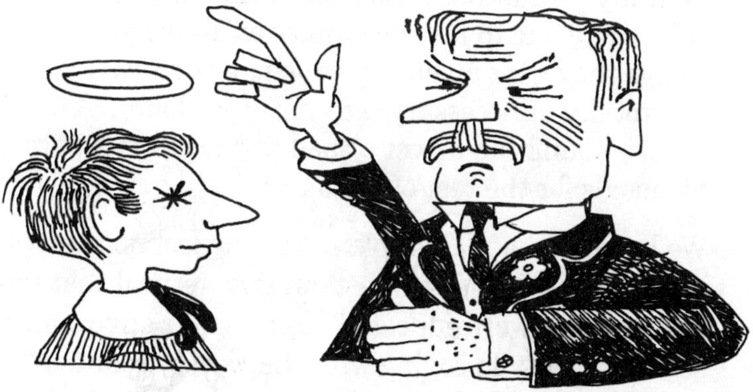

I was a young child in the early 1920s, and I learned from my father that civilization had already collapsed, and that there was no hope for the future. He was rather old when I was born, and it seemed to me that he had never come to terms with the twentieth century but judged everything by Victorian standards. Thus I learned that by the 1920s mothers no longer bothered to look after their children as they were concerned only with going to dance-halls and the cinema, that children no longer learnt anything in school as the young teachers were virtually uneducated and there was no discipline, that all younger workmen were utterly lazy and did not know their jobs, that everyone in public office was now utterly corrupt, that 'the young' no longer had any respect for their elders.

It was only much later I learned that there are records of this firm conviction existing among many older people in every century, and that it is expressed in an ancient Egyptian papyrus. It amuses me nowadays when I hear some greybeard giving vent to opinions about 'the young' identical with those of my father, to reflect that he too has once committed what William Pitt called 'The atrocious crime of being a young man', and that he may even have been one of the irresponsible youngsters that my father disapproved of so heartily.

That my poor father's indifferent health and recurrent dyspepsia was partly due to his encounters with 'the young' and the kind of things they kept inventing which he perceived as being dangerous and totally unnecessary, was never in doubt. A brush with a cheeky young cab-driver or bad service from a pert shop-girl spoilt his meals for the rest of the day.

We have here a real problem. As our technological society is developing in an exponential fashion it is natural that those of us who grew up and were educated in an earlier environment will find some difficulty in coping with the world around us as it now exists. We have grounds for envying 'the young' for their expertise with more modern machines such as computers, and we may prefer to run our lives on more simple lines, questioning whether it is necessary to clutter our homes with all sorts of electronic gadgets. Manners are changing, and it may slightly irk us that bank clerks now greet us with 'Hallo' instead of 'Good morning'. Some older people are literally frightened of the modern world and deeply distrust such things as genetic engineering, the use of contraceptive pills, designer drugs, the irradiation of food, and such distrust can become magnified into a harmful paranoia that undermines the health.

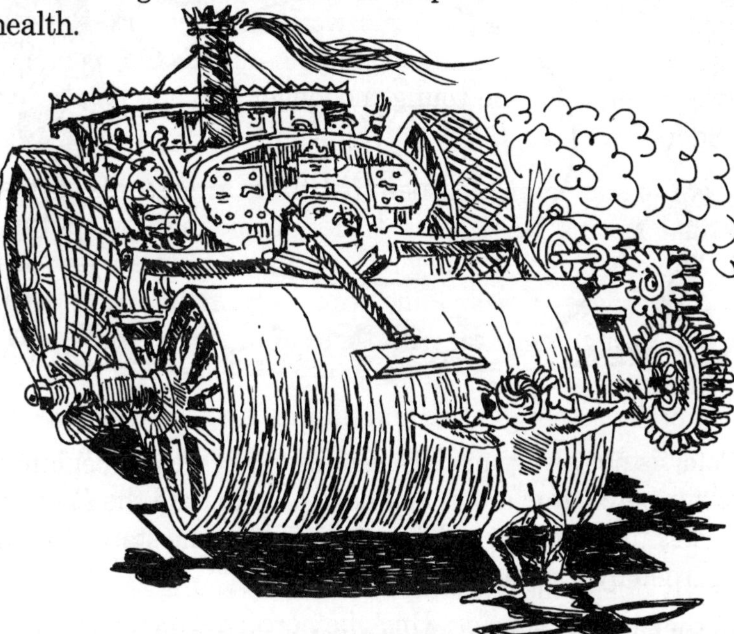

Certainly there are grave risks attendant on the introduction of all new techniques, as was pointed out when they began to use steam-power, but there is a difference between a reasonable scepticism about new developments combined with a willingness to take some risks, and a conviction that we are living perpetually on the brink of disaster that so bedevilled my poor father.

It is my thesis that in order to live happily and healthily you should be prepared to take risks, and take them having informed yourself of what the odds are as far as is possible. Being 'old' is indeed a challenge, but in the long run it is better to live boldly in the modern world rather than to shrink from it, and to have confidence in your judgement that 'a little of what you fancy does you good'.

Chapter 2

GETTING UNALIKE AS WE GET OLDER

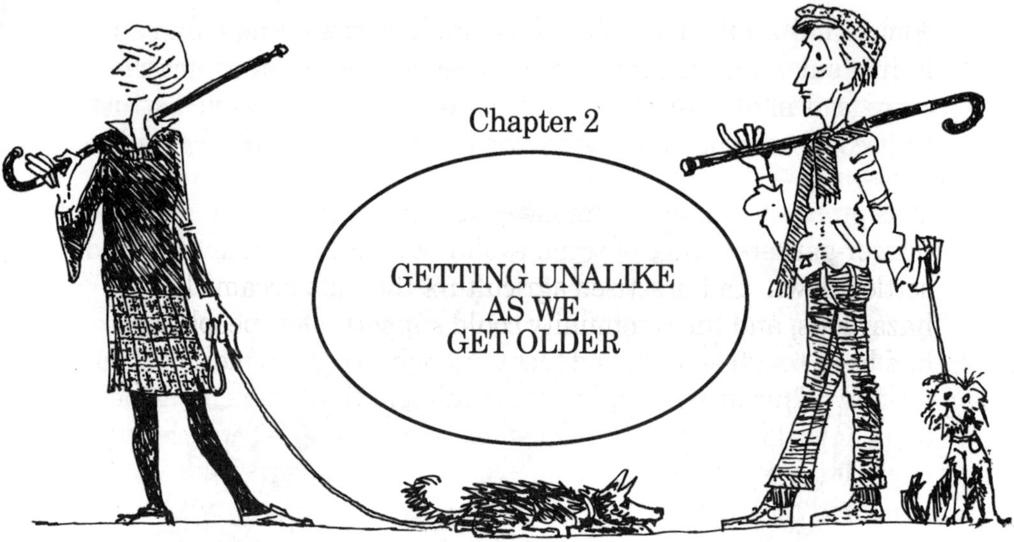

BEING OLD

Being 'old' is not a very modern condition but we are beginning to change our perception of it. You have only to read the *Book of Ecclesiastes* to encounter a description of how the state of 'oldness' was regarded by the ancient Hebrews:

Remember now thy creator in the days of thy youth, while the evil days come not, nor the years draw nigh, when thou shalt say, I have no pleasure in them.

There follows a grim description of the horrors of later life, all couched in poetic and allegorical language, making it plain why they will be evil days and old people take no pleasure in them. Ancient medical writers such as Hippocrates dwelt in some detail on the various unpleasant disabilities that attended old age, and the ugly stereotype of elderly people has come down to us through the ages. It is only in the 20th century that the condition of people in later life has improved quite dramatically, and it is now quite wrong and unnecessary that they should say, as in *Ecclesiastes*, 'I have no pleasure' in the later years.

Among most animals in the wild state it is quite rare to find an individual who is noticeably older than the other adults, for their conditions of life are generally so dangerous that any one past its prime will soon be killed off by one of the many natural hazards.

This probably applied to our early ancestors when we were at the hunter-gatherer stage of social evolution, but as soon as mankind settled down and practised agriculture then life became less hazardous, and the community could support a few people who had been tough enough and lucky enough to outlive most of their fellows. Thus in any primitive agricultural tribe there are generally a few old men and women who are not capable of much active work, but because of their long experience are tolerated or honoured for their reputed wisdom.

Even in advanced Western societies where great strides had been made in public health and nutrition, at the beginning of the 20th century, 'old' people were by no means common. In 1901 the average life expectancy at birth in the UK was only 45 years, but such enormous progress has been made during this century that by 1988 the life expectancy at birth was 71.5 years for men and 77.4 years for women. At present, about 15% of the population are past the age of retirement, a statutory age that is absurdly at variance with the difference between the sexes, because women live about six years longer than men on average.

When you read of the expectation of life at birth being only about 40 before this century, it may give the false impression that there were no long-lived people in ancient times. The fact is that the average length of life was brought down by the high mortality rate among children, and a lot of young and middle-aged adults met untimely deaths by the many infectious diseases that were around. However, those who were exceptionally tough, and extremely lucky, did live on to quite advanced ages. The records of ancient Greece that we have tell us of men who lived vigorously into old age. Isocrates, the famous Greek orator, committed suicide at the age of 98; Agesilaus, King of Sparta, although small, mean and lame, died in his 80s whilst leading a military campaign; Plato lived to the age of 81, and Sophocles died at 89, having recently been charged by his son as being of unsound mind because of his age. The judges who examined him pronounced him to be perfectly sound in mind. The fact is that there were people of advanced age living in these early societies despite their many health hazards and absence of advanced medical care, just as there are today in undeveloped countries, but in contrast to the developed countries of today, there were comparatively few of them.

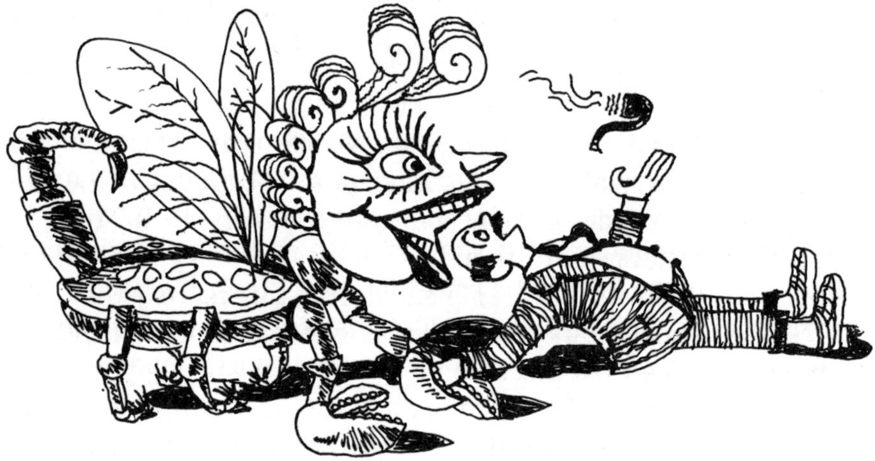

NUMERICAL EXCESS OF WOMEN

Apropos of the preponderance of women in the older years – there are twice as many by the age of 75 – the great nineteenth century French naturalist Fabre noted that most of the insects he found were female, and he wondered why. Eventually he discovered that this was due to the frequent practice of the female insects eating their mates after they had served their turn. Perhaps a similar sort of phenomenon occurs in the human species – although not literally of course. I was intrigued to find that a later natural historian, K D Roeder, writing in the *Biological Bulletin,* reported that he had found that removal of the head of the male praying mantis improved its sexual performance. This is because in this insect the subeosophageal ganglion, which is under the head, normally inhibits the copulatory movement of the abdomen. We may observe in humans that once a man has 'lost his head' over a woman he becomes a far more ardent lover, and many wives will attest that after they have 'bitten the head off' their mates a few times they become much more docile husbands!

There are many theories as to why women live longer than men, and I hasten to add that we should not generalize from insects to humans too closely, for it is found that married men live longer than unmarried men. The plain fact is that in later life women are much tougher than men, both physically and emotionally; men who lose their wives by bereavement have an increased chance of dying in the first year of their mourning, and as heart disease is one of the most frequent causes of death among men, they may be said to die of a broken heart. Women do not react thus when widowed so frequently, and some modern writers maintain that in later life women are all the better for losing their husbands. Such surveys of the opinions of widows as have been done show that nowadays the majority of widows do not wish to re-marry, but are content to go on living on their own. Whether or not they opt for taking on a 'toy boy' or other visiting lover is a matter of personal taste, chance, and circumstances.

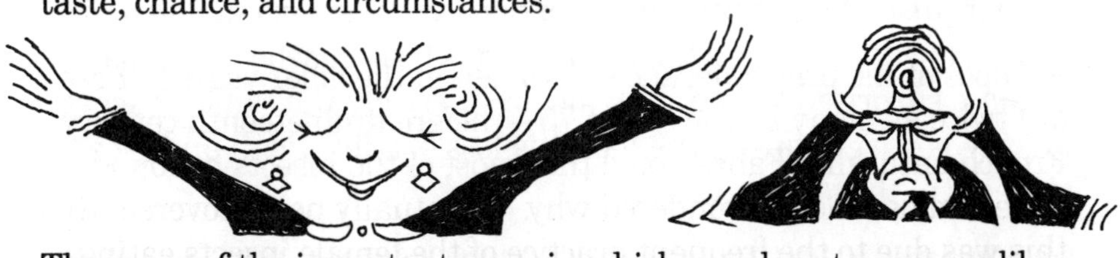

Thus, one of the important ways in which people get more unalike as they get older is that the two sexes become increasingly different in terms of robustness. It is generally assumed that women are the 'weaker sex', but in later life the traditional position is reversed.

ARE YOU AN 'OLDIE'?

When addressing some of their older patients, doctors have occasionally found that they have to be careful not to offend them by the terms they use. A surprisingly large number of such people will be slightly offended if they are referred to as 'elderly' or 'old'. The unthinking reference to 'An old lady like you . . .' may be displeasing to a woman in her sixties who does not think of herself as 'An old lady'.

In one survey 320 men and women in the age groups of the 60s, 70s and 80s were asked how they would classify themselves with respect to their age-status, and while 172 referred to themselves as 'elderly' or 'old', 148 saw themselves as 'young' or 'middle-aged'. How such a question is posed makes quite a lot of difference, but it was clear that some of them, even in the oldest, did not regard themselves as being 'old'.

Do you regard yourself as being 'old', and if so, at what age did you begin to think of yourself thus? Even if you do not now think of yourself in these terms, or as someone to whom some rude younger people might apply the derogatory slang terms 'wrinkly' or 'crumbly', is there an age in the future you envisage being in this category? Perhaps it is a question you have never bothered to think about, or perhaps at some time in the past you thought that at your present age you would be a quite different person – an oldie. Now that date on the calendar has been reached, you may be quite surprised to find that you are precisely the same – except for, say, some greying of the hair, the loss of a few teeth and greater stiffness of the joints.

WHO ARE THE OLD?

It is of interest to see just how the men and women in the study I have mentioned arrived at their judgement as to whether they were 'old' or not, and a summary of their reasons is given in the Table below:

REASONS GIVEN FOR PERSONAL AGE IDENTIFICATION IRRESPECTIVE OF ACTUAL AGE

Young or **middle-aged**	
Still active and busy	59.8%
Good physical/mental health	59.1%
Positive mental attitude	28.9%
Rapport with young people	14.1%
Youthful appearance	8.4%
Mix with all ages	8.4%
Handles own affairs	7.0%
Other	7.0%
Elderly or **old**	
Health problem, e.g. heart attack	28.5%
Retirement	22.1%
Physical slowdown, e.g. tire easily	20.3%
Health restrictions	12.8%
'Just age' (no other reason)	11.6%
Change in social contacts	5.8%
Illness or death of spouse	5.8%
Other	15.1%

These figures have been taken from *The Aging Experience* by Russell A Ward (1979), by kind permission of the author and the publishers HarperCollins.

It will be seen that the most important reasons for people regarding themselves as 'young' or 'middle-aged' irrespective of their actual age, were concerned with physical and psychological health, and as 'elderly' or 'old' also concerned health or the fact of retirement. Thus, sickly men or women in their early 60s, who have retired from work and have no particular occupation, may regard themselves as 'elderly or old', whereas healthy people in their 80s who are still busily occupied, either gainfully or voluntarily, may still see themselves as no more than 'middle-aged', and may indeed have long ago given up bothering about their age.

Occasionally, someone in their 80s may say that when they attend gatherings of retired people, some rather younger than themselves, they look around at the grey heads and wrinkled faces, and think to themselves, 'Poor old things – I'm glad I'm not like them!' Have you ever had this experience? Simone de Beauvoir observed that 'old people are also mirrors for one another, mirrors in which they do not care to see themselves – the marks of old age they behold vex them'. The viewer sees the externals, and because of long conditioning by society's stereotypes of age, cannot realize that many of these people feel just like they do in their inner selves.

The fact that someone looks 'old' and is indeed a very senior citizen according to the date of birth, does not mean that he or she is in any way different, intellectually, emotionally or socially, from younger people. Much depends upon the individual. Although I have just discussed how health determines, to some extent, people's perception of themselves with respect to age-status, health is a relative matter. One can be sickly at any age, yet still feel and act vigorously intellectually and emotionally. The fact that some people in the last decades of their life take up totally new careers, develop fresh and absorbing interests, fall in love, and give other signs of that intangible quality of a 'positive mental attitude', as mentioned in the Table above, is evidence that the potential for living life to the full need not evaporate with age.

The question of subjective age in relation to chronological age has been discussed in some detail in order to indicate the difficulty in referring to 'the elderly', or using other such labels. In this book I will use such terms as 'older people' or 'people in later life' without being too definite as to the chronological milestones indicated. The term the Third Age is generally used of those who have retired from full-time work by reason of their age, but the age of retirement is determined by law and may be changed. It is a flexible thing, and varies between occupations – some academics are allowed to keep their jobs for two years after the statutory age.

Within this Third Age there is a huge variation between individuals as to health status, their fitness for work, and their self-perception of 'oldness'. This variation is determined by three things: their genetic potential that was determined at the moment of conception, their life history in terms of health, and how they are regarded by the society in which they live.

1. **Genetic Potential.**

Many features of your future life were determined at the moment of your conception by your genetic potential, although of course in most things, what you have actually become has been the result of an interaction between potential and environmental forces such as education, health etc. Environment would not alter pre-determined things like the colour of your eyes, and within limits, your height. You might have been a little shorter if you had been malnourished in youth, but you have your ancestors to thank for most aspects of your physical body. There are some changes that take place in later life that appear to be programmed to happen and that nothing can alter; thus the sad condition of Huntington's Chorea does not show itself typically until after the age of 40; up to that age the individual appears to be normal, but once it has become manifest the individual has only about 15 more years to live. Programming is not usually as definite as that, but a number of conditions such as Alzheimer's disease probably have a genetic basis in some, if not all cases, although certain environmental conditions which are not yet understood may produce the disease in later life in those who are susceptible.

Just as some individuals are destined to be tall and others to be short (assuming adequate nutrition and health) so it is possible that some are programmed to live much longer than others, and that there is very little that we can do about it, other than behave in a way to secure the optimum of health. You may have noted that among your friends and members of your family, some have died at an age rather younger than you expected, and you may have felt almost guilty, thinking, 'Oh dear, if only we had persuaded him not to emigrate, not to marry that awful woman, not to have gone in for farming, not to have become a teetotaller (etc., etc.) he might have been alive today'. Such self-recriminations may be totally unnecessary, for we do not know what leads to a long or short life-span, except that maintaining general health is about the best we can do, and the rules for health are really very simple.

One of the most striking differences between people that become manifest with age concerns their robustness. The difference is so very much against commonly accepted beliefs as this quote from a very eminent specialist in the study of ageing, Dr Grimley Evans, states:

> There are no discontinuities in later life that could provide a biological justification for separating the elderly from the rest of the adult human race. Moreover, we age at different rates, so that inter-individual variance increases with age. Although on average functional abilities decline with age, some individuals aged 80 will still be performing within the normal range of 30 year-old people.

Unquestionably, the 80-year-olds who are performing as though they were in their 30s have led very healthy lives, and have been lucky in escaping accidents, but it seems likely that such exceptional people have been genetically programmed to be long-lived, and if we inquired into their ancestry it would be apparent that they came of a long-lived family.

Longevity in humans is a very complex matter: in some animal species breeding experiments have shown that a single gene has a powerful effect on the animal's life-span, but although it is not feasible to carry out breeding experiments with humans, such evidence as we have indicates that in humans the life-span is determined 'polygenetically', that is, a number of different genes determine our potential longevity.

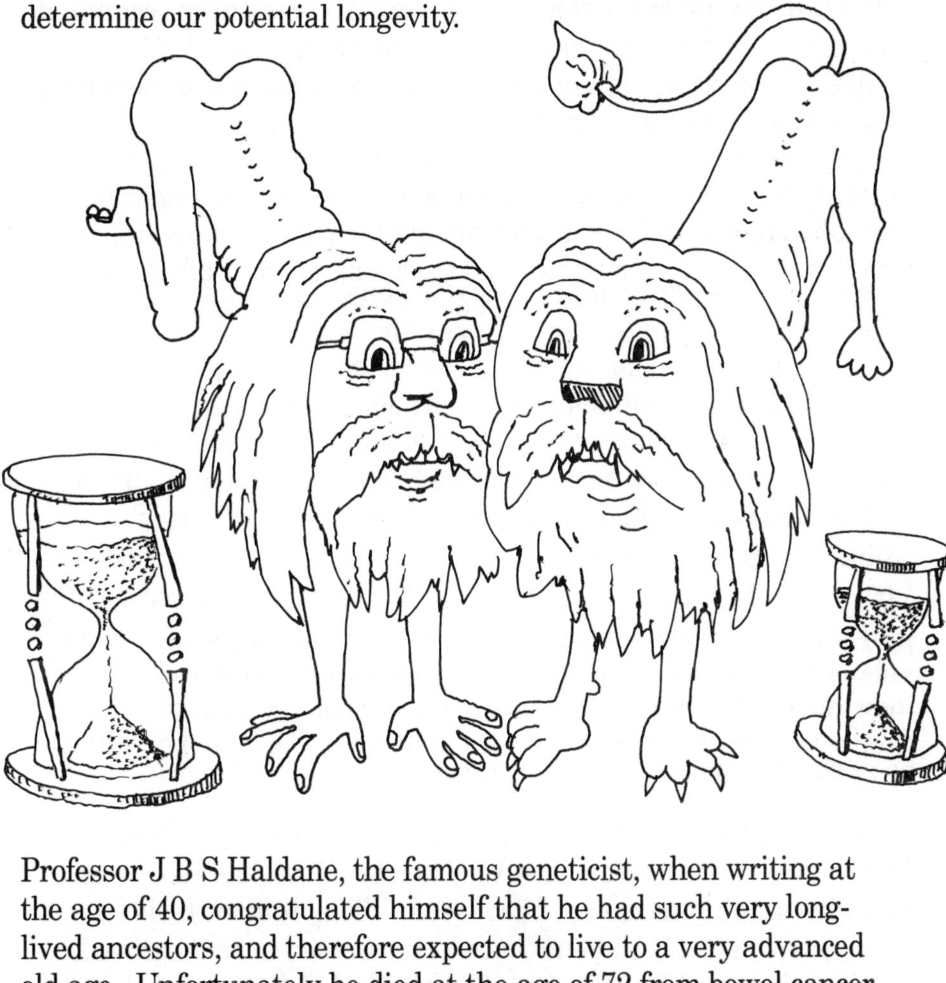

Professor J B S Haldane, the famous geneticist, when writing at the age of 40, congratulated himself that he had such very long-lived ancestors, and therefore expected to live to a very advanced old age. Unfortunately he died at the age of 72 from bowel cancer. It may have been that among his genes was a predisposition to cancer (a disease that we still know rather little about) or perhaps environmental factors determined that the cancer would develop for reasons quite unconnected with his genetic endowment.

When discussing longevity we need to be careful not to confuse cause with effect. I used to know a lady who was very vigorous in her 90s and she boasted that her long life and energy were due to the curious vegetarian diet she lived on. When someone commented on her obvious toughness, another friend responded, 'Yes, Lilian's strong, very tough – you'd need to be exceptionally tough to live on the muck she eats!'

2. **Life History**

Factors in your early life may have an effect on your health when you are old. There is some evidence that diet and other life-style influences on a pregnant mother may affect the foetus, so that later on such an individual may be vulnerable to certain diseases that affect subsequent longevity. Whether the mother refrained from smoking, drank only moderately and had a decent mixed diet during pregnancy will have a long-term effect on her offspring throughout their future lives. Those who are now in their 50s are benefiting from the wise provision of free orange juice, cod-liver oil and milk to infants during the period of rationing during and after the war. The disease of rickets in childhood, which is due to lack of adequate calcium in the diet and insufficiency of Vitamin D, will have a long-term effect on the skeleton and make the individual vulnerable to diseases of the bones in later life.

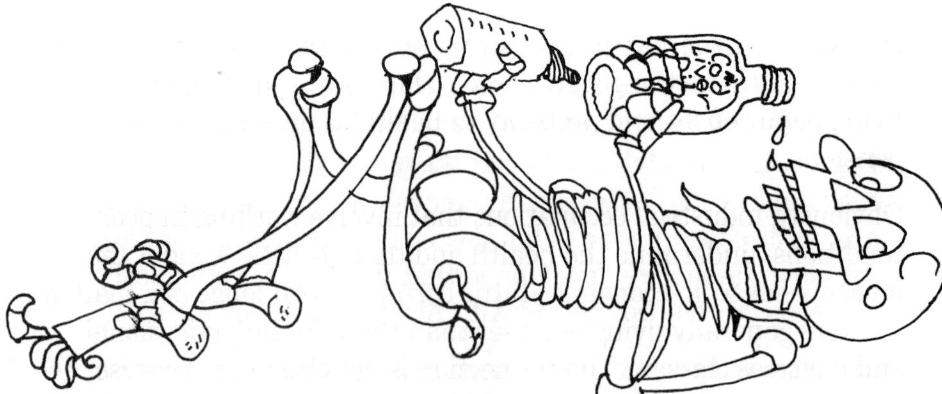

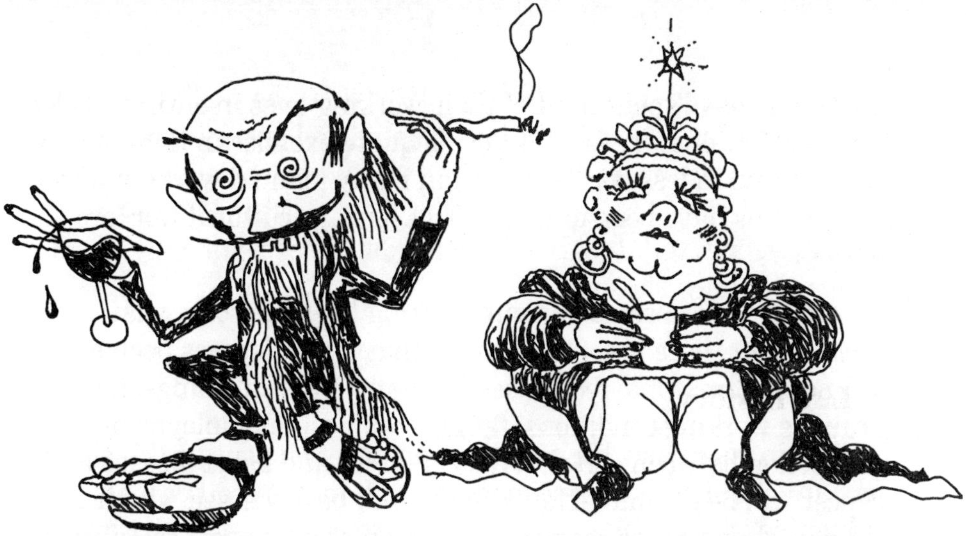

The habits you have acquired during the course of your life, such as smoking, drinking too much and eating an unwise diet, may result in various disabilities in the later years. Fortunately it is never too late to change unsuitable habits however old you are; giving up smoking will prevent further risk of damage to the lungs and heart, and adopting a life-style that embraces adequate exercise will contribute to reducing a tendency to obesity with all its consequent ills, including diabetes.

Life history includes both education and occupation. Those who have been better educated enjoy a double advantage: first, they are more able to appreciate the benefits of a healthy life-style and to know how best to deal with the health hazards of life; second, as education is generally linked with economic security they are less likely to fall into the poverty trap in later life and be reduced to living penuriously, and probably unhealthily, on a wretched pension.

Obviously, industrial occupations that involve working in poor conditions, undermine the health and there is little wonder that measures of socio-economic status correlate with longevity, manual workers generally dying younger than those in the professional and business classes. The connection is not clear-cut of course, as those who have spent most of their working lives in entirely sedentary occupations without taking adequate exercise in their leisure time end up in less good shape than many manual workers whose occupations have been quite healthy, like agricultural workers and gardeners.

The effects of stress during our working lives are somewhat unclear, but there is some evidence that it predisposes people to sickness. Stress may be caused by many different things including arduous working conditions, family troubles, unemployment. The connection between certain types of stress and heart disease and cancer will be examined later, and it will be discussed whether therapy that aims to reduce stress, even at a late age, can counter a predisposition to heart attacks and cancer.

3. **How society regards the ageing individual**

The health status of people in the Third Age is determined not only by their individual genetic predispositions and the sort of lives they have led, but also by the way society as a whole regards them. If a society regards its senior citizens as a nuisance and a burden on scarce medical and social resources it will affect their health materially.

First, the provisions for pensions and social services for the old will be somewhat meagre and, second, the elderly people themselves will be made to feel unwanted and expected to go cap-in-hand when they claim what is their statutory right, with a permanent sense of anxiety that what they already receive may be reduced or withdrawn. This diffident attitude accounts for the fact that, according to the Department of Social Security, in one year 900,000 pensioners failed to claim the benefits to which they were entitled, and this applied principally to Supplementary Benefit – 79% of elderly and impoverished pensioners failed to claim it.

It may be that many frail older people fail to ask for the benefits to which they are entitled because they do not realize that the various ailments from which they suffer are not the inevitable consequences of ageing, but are perfectly remedial by appropriate medical and social measures.

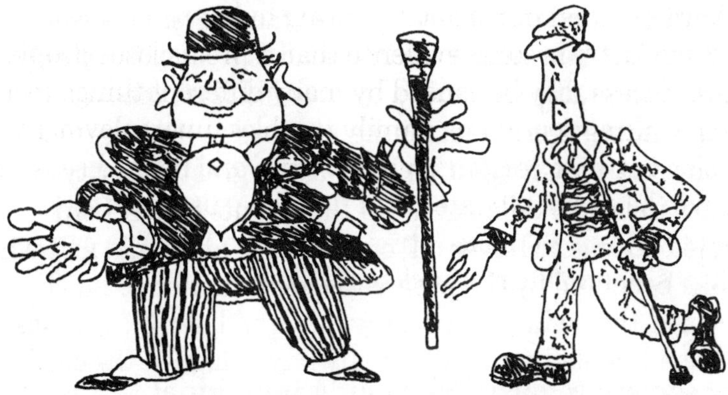

Here we have a sad paradox: those who are most in need are generally the most timid – they are the frail, impoverished, ill-educated working-class pensioners. People who are better educated and who have a proper sense of their own importance are not so diffident in standing up for their rights and demanding the share of the cake that is lawfully due to them.

There are welcome signs that the 'new old' as they are sometimes called – people who have retired more recently – do have a better appreciation of their own value and their right to health and happiness, and are not prepared to live in the shadow on the margins of society. Partly as a consequence of their greater determination to look after themselves their health is indeed better than that of their parents and grandparents at an equivalent age. They are less likely to put up with deteriorating quietly from chronic pathological conditions, and thus, paradoxically, although they will live longer they will be less of a burden on the medical and social services in the long run.

ARE YOU 'WALKING WOUNDED'
OR A 'SEASONED SURVIVOR'?

There is some debate at present whether the people who are now becoming 'old' in terms of their date of birth, will be especially frail or especially robust later on. The argument goes like this: as medical practice and public health have made great strides in efficiency in the last half-century, will it lead to a lot of the chronically infirm and vulnerable who previously would have died off in middle-age, now lingering on for many years as an increased burden on society? Or will it be that as the great majority of people now in late middle-age were the infants whom Lord Woolton fed on free cod-liver oil, orange juice and milk, and whose health has benefited by the progressive elimination of much childhood disease, they will be especially tough in later life and resistant to the ailments that traditionally have plagued the old?

I have labelled the former type 'Walking Wounded' and the latter 'Seasoned Survivors'. Some people may object to my arbitrarily dividing people into two groups like this, but while admitting that it is an over-simplification, it will serve to illustrate the sort of difference I wish to discuss.

The Walking Wounded

The 'walking wounded' are those who by genetic endowment, or by living a most unhealthy life, or by a combination of both, arrive at their Third Age in pretty bad shape. In stringent circumstances, such as exist in some third world countries, they might have never reached the Third Age but died in middle age, but with the care that is available in most advanced countries they may certainly enter the Third Age. Even though they may have rather low resistance to disease, nowadays they benefit from the modern techniques of immunization against influenza and pneumonia.

It is never too late to take yourself in hand; if you are a 'walking wounded' you should observe all sensible precautions, such as are advised in this book and specially beware of becoming that terrible thing – a hypochondriac. If you keep on going to your doctor needlessly, it will be no wonder if your GP does not take your complaints quite as seriously as those of other patients. Some of the 'walking wounded' live to a ripe old age and quite enjoy life and a few of them – if they can get people to listen to them – may be said literally to 'enjoy ill health'.

The Seasoned Survivors

The 'seasoned survivors' do not necessarily enter the Third Age complete and unscarred. Having survived the long battle of life they may have various things wrong with them, but they have learned how to live with and overcome their disabilities. An extraordinary finding of research is that as far as longevity goes subjective health, that is, the way you feel 'in yourself', is more predictive than medically determined health.

Someone may have all sorts of things wrong with them that show up on careful medical examination and testing, but they feel quite fit and act as though they were quite well, and that is what is important to the enjoyment of life, and indeed, to its long continuance. I hasten to add that the results of medical examination should not be ignored: the doctor will know which signs are important and will institute further testing if anything sinister shows up that needs immediate treatment. Conditions such as a hiatus hernia or diverticulosis are so common in later life that they hardly need attention if the patient feels comfortable with them.

So the 'seasoned survivor' need take no further notice of health matters? Not at all; you should not push your luck but take active steps to maintain your health and wellbeing, with due consideration of all the added hazards of later life that you must be prepared to cope with.

THE RIGHT TO BE DIFFERENT

This chapter has explored all the many ways in which people become more different from one another as they age, and you should consider just what style of life suits you best. Unfortunately in the latter half of the twentieth century the enormous differences between people in later life are in danger of being overlooked and it seems that it is 'politically correct' to assume that we are all as alike as peas in a pod. The media frequently refers to 'the elderly' as if these millions of people were an homogenous mass. It has become almost indecent to acknowledge that innate differences in potential due to genetic differences exist right from the moment of conception, for the modern zeitgeist is to pretend that all differences are due to environmental factors and to act accordingly.

The enormous differences between people in later life are ignored, note our statutory retirement age. As one geriatrician writes of retirement rather bitterly:

> At this age they 'retire', or in plain words, are rendered unemployed, useless and, in some cases, impoverished. After that transition, and in proportion with their chronological age, they are prescribed to be unintelligent, unemployable, crazy and asexual.

There are several reasons for the modern drive to ignore individual differences between people, and to pretend that you are just like your neighbour because you happen to be of the same chronological age. One important factor is a real confusion between our equal rights as citizens, and our unequal capacities and needs. According to the Christian church we are all 'equal in the sight of God', which is a perfectly fair concept, but according to the 19th century hymn:

The rich man in his castle,

The poor man at his gate

God made them, high or lowly,

And order'd their estate.

As the 'estate' of man was supposed to be divinely ordained, he would have to wait until after his death before any recognition of his equality would occur. A strong reaction against this attempt to keep the poor in their place has characterized the present century, and has led to the confusion between rights and capacities.

Another factor leading to a genuine ignorance about the realities of inborn individual differences is the smallness of the family unit. When people had large families they were made aware that their many children, reared under identical circumstances, would show very different capacities and might have quite different needs. Now with there being only two or three in the family, parents are apt to believe that all the differences between their children and their eventual careers are determined entirely by their upbringing and the general environmental influences around them. It has become heresy to suggest that they might benefit from very different types of schooling.

Writing in 1932 and looking forwards to a better future Professor Haldane took the view of education that most informed people had at that time:

Today we often have special schools for mentally deficient children, and occasionally for very able ones. This system will, *of course,* be greatly extended. When children of all grades were combined in one class the intelligent merely learn to be lazy while the stupid are hopelessly discouraged. And the attempt to remedy this defect by placing children of widely different ages in the same class is also a failure.

Haldane was a socialist and a great champion of equality of

individual rights to fulfil their individual potential; I have italicized the words 'of course' to draw attention to his confidence and calm expectation of a more enlightened future. He was too optimistic; he was not to know what was to come towards the end of the century.

This digression into considering education has been necessary as an example of the muddle we are in today. It is important for the sake of your health and happiness that you should seriously consider how your individual needs and capacities are not necessarily the same as all people of your age. You are not just 'an oldie' – you are *you*.

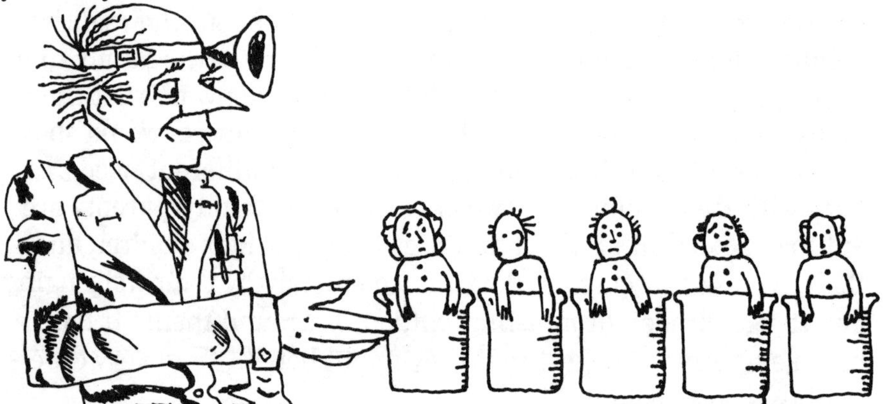

Healthcare professionals as a body have been trained in the modern climate of assuming that all people over a certain age are to be lumped together as having the same problems and needs, but their more progressive colleagues are at pains to criticize this assumption. I respect orthodox medical practice, yet at the same time I insist that in some cases the patient knows best what is good for himself or herself.

If, at the age of 80 you are habitually brisk and active, and have no problems with mobility, and you suddenly find that, perhaps after a short illness, you lose your accustomed energy and have to lie down for two hours every afternoon, your complaint may not be treated sufficiently seriously by a doctor who is not experienced in geriatric medicine. Such a doctor may look at your date of birth and then say something like, 'Well, it's just your age; you must learn to take it easy'. Such a diagnosis of 'old age' should not be accepted; if you know yourself to be normally active and energetic, a sudden loss of energy should be indicative of the beginning of a number of serious conditions, and should immediately be investigated by the various medical techniques that are now available. If they show nothing – well and good; you will just have to struggle on to regain your energy by every sensible means possible, reviewing your whole life-style.

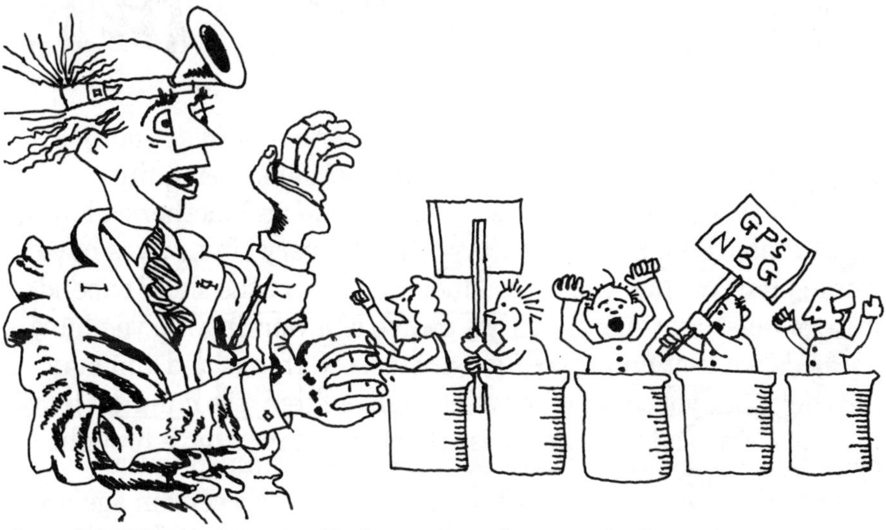

Age should not necessarily be accepted as an explanatory cause. But faced with the enormous range of differences in the health-status of patients between the ages of 30 and 80, as emphasised by Dr Grimley Evans, the inexperienced doctor is indeed in a dilemma, as discussed in Chapter 6.

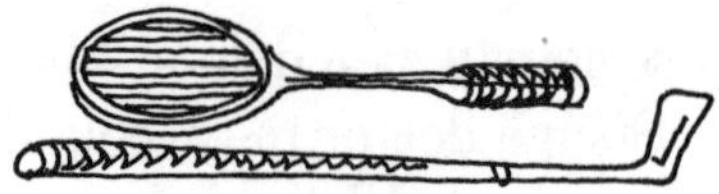

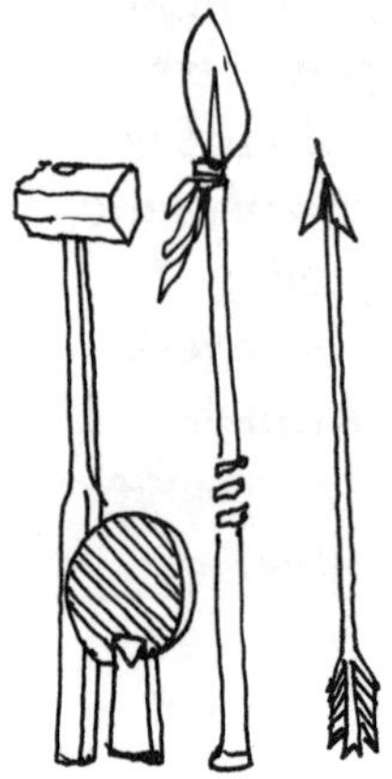

Chapter 3

HOW MUCH EXERCISE DO YOU TAKE?

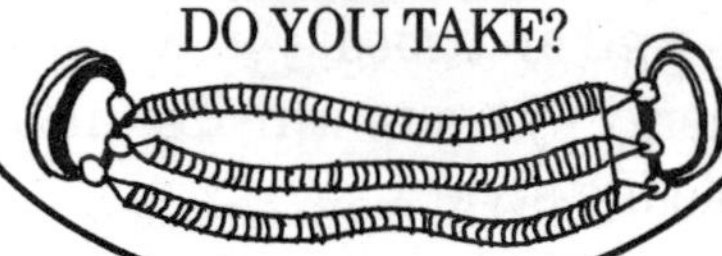

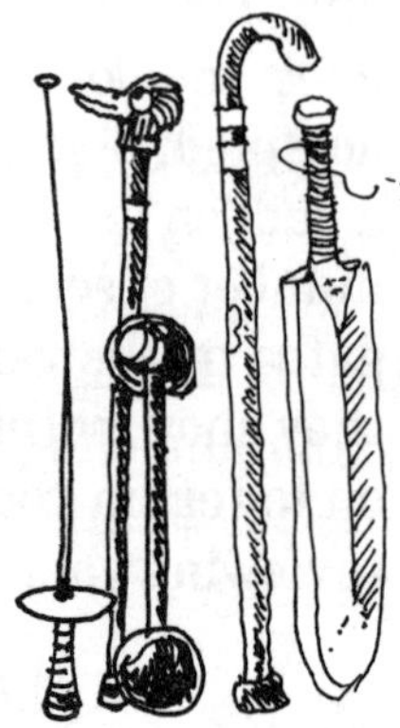

For most of your life you have probably worked hard at your job, borne the strain of daily travelling, and perhaps been quite energetic at sports. The tasks of a housewife and mother call for a considerable amount of physical work, and very often wives have worked harder than their husbands in terms of the sheer expenditure of muscular energy. In the course of a working life you have learned that rest and relaxation are blessed things and you may have felt that you couldn't have enough of them; the children leaving home was sad in a way, bless them, but it may have brought you a new lease of life.

Now you have retired you have plenty of opportunity for rest, but how much of it does you good? You don't have to work, but as a reaction from your previous energetic and even over-worked life, perhaps you are taking just too much rest. That square box in the sittingroom and the deck chair in the garden, even the comfortable chairs in the local pub may be doing you no good at all. The question of the proper amount of exercise you should take for the benefit of your general health and your continued fitness was one of the questions investigated in the Carnegie Third Age Inquiry.

The mere fact of ageing results in a decline of physical fitness and you take it for granted that at the age of 60 you cannot run round the block as quickly as you did when you were aged 25; this fact of life does not worry you. But few people realize how early in life the decline begins. For averagely fit men at the age of 25, walking uphill (1 in 7 gradient) requires just a moderate effort from the heart muscle, but this effort increases steadily throughout life, so that by the age of 65 walking up hills of this gradient requires maximum effort of the heart. If we turn to the study of people who are 'unfit', and we can be less than fit at any age, at age 25 walking uphill requires severe effort from the heart, and by the age of 65 may be impossible. Here, of course, I am talking about averages, and as elsewhere in this book I must stress that as we get older we get more and more unalike one another, so that by the age of 65 a few people are like those ten years younger than their actual age.

This individual variation in the rate and extent of decline is governed by two factors: first, our genetic programming; some of us are destined to be vigorous up to extreme old age and this is entirely a matter of the genes we have inherited; second, our environment and behaviour, play their part – the sort of life we have lived in our earlier years, including situations that could result in accident or disease, and the life-style we continue to adhere to in later life. It will be appreciated therefore, that even if we have not been particularly fortunate in the parents we picked, we can do a great deal about determining how healthy we shall be by conscious planning. Fortunately it is never too late to modify our way of living and benefit from it.

First I will describe what can be called the 'natural' decline with ageing, the processes we can't do much about, and then I will describe the sorts of decline that are due to unwise behaviour, and in this chapter I will concentrate on the role of exercise in maintaining health. We now have the benefit of a great deal of research that has gone into this matter, serving to discredit some of the old wives' tales that we grew up with, and are still believed by quite a number of people.

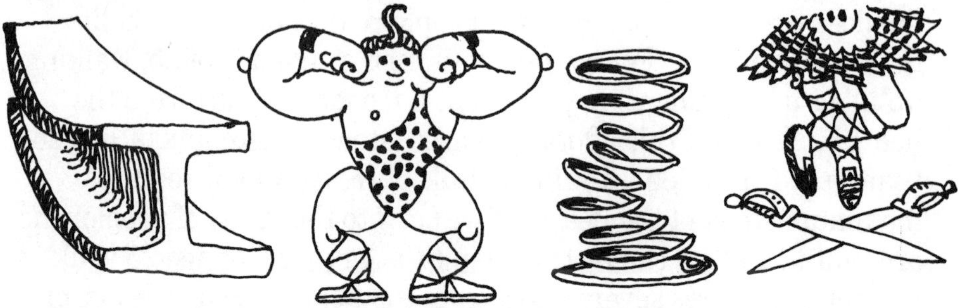

THE DETERMINANTS OF PHYSICAL FITNESS

It is useful to consider physical fitness in terms of four attributes: stamina, strength, suppleness and skill.

Stamina

Stamina refers to the ability to sustain activity, and it is dependent on the rate at which the muscles and other tissues can use oxygen that is supplied by the blood-stream. This assumes, of course, that the body is being supplied with adequate nutrients which are the 'fuel' used for work. As there is a natural decline in the working efficiency of the heart and lungs with age, so stamina is reduced, and we cannot go on working or exercising, without increasingly longer periods of rest. There are other complex factors involved, and there is also a loss of the sheer bulk of muscles as we age which makes physical tasks more effortful.

Strength

As we age so the muscles very gradually waste in bulk, and after the age of about 60 this process is accelerated, so that by the age of 70 muscle-power is reduced by about 20%. Unfortunately the muscles of the lower limbs that are important for walking are particularly vulnerable, a finding that give some confirmation to Shakespeares picture of the sixth age of man:

. . . the lean and slippered pantaloon,

With spectacles on nose and pouch on side,

His youthful hose well saved a world too wide

For his shrunk shank . . .

The muscle-power of the upper limbs also declines, and it has been estimated that this begins to fade from about the age of 40. Naturally the hazards to older people such as stumbling and falling are increased by deterioration of the general strength of the muscles and the lengthening of reaction-time with age.

Suppleness

From after the age of about 30 onwards our bodies become less supple, which is largely due to very gradual deterioration of the joints. This is hardly noticeable in most people as middle-age advances, but in later life it may become a very definite problem, and is known as 'Osteoarthritis'. These degenerative changes are not limited to the joints only; tendons, ligaments and muscles are affected. Muscles slowly lose their bulk and power with age, but they are also subject to a growing stiffness. In youth you were probably conscious of how stiff your muscles might become the day after you had engaged in violent exercise, but in later life this stiffness comes more after prolonged lack of use rather than activity.

Skill

Of the four attributes of physical fitness skill is perhaps the most difficult clearly to define. You may generally associate skill with learned abilities such as playing the piano, writing, talking, driving a car, riding a bicycle and the skills of crafts such as cabinet-making, dressmaking, etc. These skills deteriorate very little with ageing, and a very elderly person may still possess them to a remarkable degree. He or she may have to abandon such occupations simply because of failing eyesight and rheumatism of the joints, but you may regard such a person as still having the skill but being unable to exercise it because of growing inability of the peripheral physical apparatus.

However, other skills that we don't normally think about are essential for the activity of daily living. We don't consciously know how we walk down stairs; we just do it 'automatically' having learned the skill in infancy.

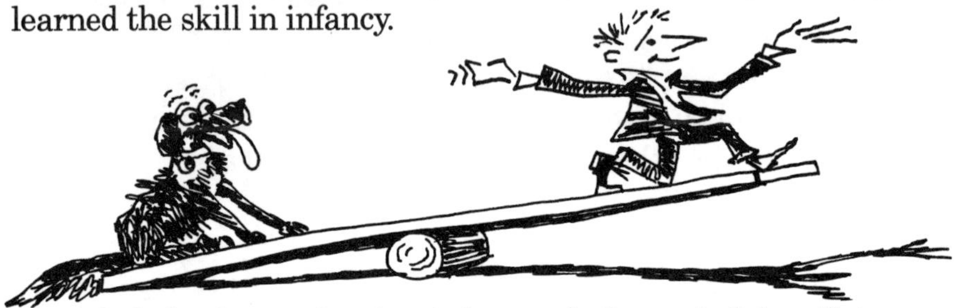

The whole business of maintaining our balance, judging distances, dressing, co-ordinating body movements, depends on a fine interplay between incoming signals from sight, hearing, proprioception (feedback from muscles and joints) and the executive action of our muscles. As sight and hearing fade with age, despite compensation by spectacles and hearing-aids, we become less steady on our legs and less sure in the delicate control of our hands, so generalized skill can be said to fade. We may become 'clumsy' in later life, and this has important implications for looking after ourselves and avoiding falls and other accidents in the home.

THE FITNESS GAP

The gradually failing health that occurs with ageing can therefore be attributed to two factors, one inevitable and the other which is both preventable and remedial, and this is shown in the following figure. It will be seen that the 'fitness gap', the distance between natural decline with ageing (dotted line) and the decline due to an incorrect life-style (solid line), gets progressively greater because the older you get the less you are able to withstand the ravages of sickness, inactivity, smoking, incorrect diet etc.

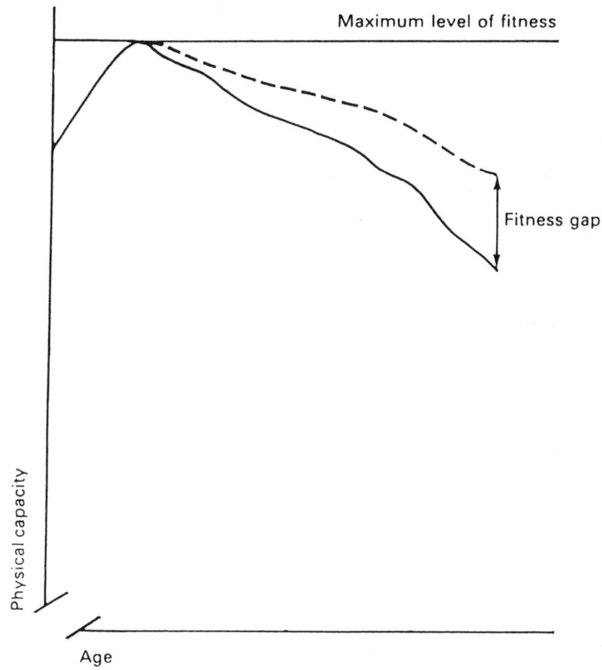

Reproduced from *Prevention of Disease in the Elderly* by kind permission of the author J A Muir Gray, and the publishers Churchill Livingstone.

WHAT YOU CAN DO ABOUT IT

I have described the various ways in which the fitness of the body declines with the normal process of ageing. You cannot alter this biological fact, but you can do a great deal to minimize the decline and compensate for it, and much of your action will depend upon how much you understand what is going on and realize your potential for looking after yourself. I shall quote one of the scientists,

Sarah Lamb, who contributed to the Carnegie Third Age Inquiry which examined the role of exercise in later life:

> A growing consensus of opinion points to the significant role that exercise has in the maintenance of physical and mental health, and functional ability . . . Despite this, on average, the fitness of individuals in the third age, and their participation in exercise, is below that required to ensure good functioning in daily life . . . This should obviously be of considerable concern to all who are involved in providing care for people in the third age.

The person who is most concerned in providing care for you is, of course, yourself. You may well say 'That's all very well, but how much exercise should I be taking? Perhaps I'm doing very nicely as I am.' I will address this question more precisely later on, but meanwhile take a look at what people say about their own health.

In the National Fitness Survey of the Sports Council and Health Education Authority people aged 55 -74 were asked to assess themselves as to their fitness, and the results of this survey are shown below.

Percentage distribution of self-assessment of fitness levels in those aged 55-74.

	Men	**Women**
Very fit	23%	26%
Fairly fit	56%	60%
Not very fit	15%	11%
Not fit at all	6%	3%

The figures seem very satisfactory, especially for the women, 86% of whom regard themselves as very or fairly fit, yet according to the researchers 'nearly all' the women in this age band would find it difficult to walk up a hill with a 5% gradient. There may be several explanations for this stark contrast between self-assessment and established fact, the most obvious being that in later life both men and women have very low expectations of what they should be capable. It may be that the past stereotypes of older people have convinced them that they are pathetic old things who should count themselves lucky if they can still stagger out to the local shops and back and that they are 'fairly fit' if they can do so. But times are changing, and it has been pointed out from many quarters that people entering the Third Age may have about 20 – 30 years of life to live, and that it should be a period of active enjoyment of a worthwhile and interesting life.

Some are questioning whether 'the old' are becoming an increasing burden on society as they are becoming more numerous. Certainly the oldest 15% of the population are estimated to consume 25% of the medical services; no-one likes to suggest that public euthanasia centres should be set up to reduce this perceived burden, but some responsible people hint at it – all in fun of course! But behind such 'funny jokes' there is perhaps a serious concern. Donald Gould, writing in the *New Scientist*, suggests the following:

> Old people don't earn any money and have to be paid a pension. They frequently suffer ills of the flesh so that their crumbling bodies clog up family doctors' waiting rooms and occupy an absurdly high proportion of costly hospital beds. Their younger relatives have better things to do than act as unpaid servants to wrinklies no longer capable of looking after themselves. In short oldies are a damned nuisance all round, and their numbers are increasing at an alarming rate . . . There have been suggestions that before too long the state will have to impose a statutory age limit on the right to life. This could involve oldsters receiving on, say, their 75th birthday, a buff OHMS envelope instructing them to attend their local euthanasia depot on the following Wednesday at 2.30 in the afternoon.

The article continues in a jocular manner suggesting ways in which 'the old' could be disposed of, and it is accompanied by a humorous cartoon to make it clear that it is not to be taken too seriously. We oldies must stand up for ourselves; if a similar jesting article had been published on the subject of the high unemployment rate of black people in our society, one can imagine the outcry there would have been. But surely it is up to the retired section of the population to see that they are as little a burden as possible, and this for our own self-respect, satisfaction and enjoyment of life.

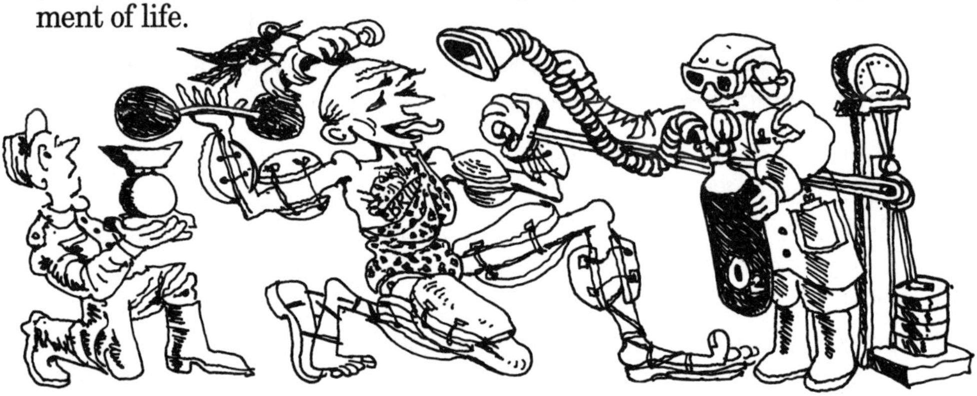

HOW FITNESS MAY BE REGAINED IN LATER LIFE

The good news is that although you may have become rather unfit for this reason or that, you can take active steps to regain a level of fitness appropriate to your age. Obviously if you suffer from medical conditions such as diabetes, gastric ulcer, emphysema, cancer, chronic heart disease, etc., etc., these conditions must be thoroughly investigated and treated medically, and the nature of these treatments is outside the scope of this book. But you may have no definite disorder or disease and still be far from as fit as you should be at your age. Whatever the reasons are for your past deterioration in health, there is no reason why you should not now take yourself in hand and implement sensible measures to improve your present status. It is very important that you should understand the nature of the remedies proposed, and be in the position of your own health expert in so far as it is up to you, and not your doctor, to look after yourself.

Improving Stamina

Stamina, the ability to continue to work or make any form of physical effort, is ultimately dependent on supplying muscles and other tissues of the body with the oxygen we extract from the air by breathing. The term 'aerobic power' is generally used to describe this, and consumption of oxygen can be measured quite easily in clinical trials.

In one scientific study of 38 people between the ages of 60 and 70 their aerobic power was measured over a period of 7 weeks during which they were participating in a programme of exercise conditioning. The scientists who conducted this study commented that:

> maximum oxygen intake was brought quite quickly to the level anticipated in a sedentary person ten to twenty years younger than the test subject.

Another study concerned 112 men aged between 52 and 88 years, and by an appropriate programme of exercises produced an improvement in the function of the heart and breathing, and thus effected a significant increase in the mechanisms by which the muscles were supplied with oxygen, and hence in their stamina.

Improving Strength

As already discussed, our muscles get weaker both by the natural process of ageing and by the various ways in which we have neglected our health, particularly by under-exercise. However, it has been demonstrated that a training programme may restore the lost strength to the muscles of men as old as 70.

In one of these studies the men were required to perform appropriate exercises three times a week for 12 weeks. The scientists took biopsies of the muscles both before and after the period of training, and demonstrated that there had been an actual increase in the bulk of the muscle-fibres. A biopsy is a process in which a minute sample of body cells is extracted for examination under the microscope, or otherwise tested. These studies showed that the increase in strength was not just a temporary phenomenon, such as might be obtained by increased motivation of the subjects, but that there had been actual growth of the muscles.

Improving suppleness

It is rather difficult to take adequate measures of joint stiffness or suppleness, nevertheless it has been done. In one study a dance-and-exercise programme was introduced, which is probably less boring than simply performing exercises, and this was done thrice weekly for 12 weeks, and it produced increased movement in six joints – neck, wrist, shoulder, hip and back, knee and ankle. The trouble about people performing exercises in their own homes, as they are often told to do by physiotherapists engaged in rehabilitation programmes after accidents is that the process becomes very boring, and people are apt to skip or curtail their exercise periods. It is much better that people should meet together in groups, and dancing or yoga exercises may be combined in a social occasion during which people give one another mutual support and encouragement.

Improving skill

It is within common experience that if you cease to exert a skill such as piano playing or typing, for a long time, you become 'rusty' in it and can no longer perform it with your previous dexterity. However, if you try to take it up again you will re-learn it far quicker than anyone who has never learnt it in the first place.

This implies that skills depend not only on the aptitude of the physical part of the body involved (e.g. the fingers) but on assemblies of cells in the brain that represent the memory for the skill. There is little evidence that any significant change takes place in the brain with ageing, so in relearning a skill it is a matter of the body getting accustomed to a pattern of impulses from the nerves that was formerly well-rehearsed. Earlier I discussed how people might become 'clumsy' in later life and less able to perform the skilful actions they used to, such as walking along a narrow plank or even dressing themselves neatly and rapidly. Much of this loss of skill is due to decreased suppleness of joints, imperfect eyesight and, most importantly, less confidence in physical ability.

If you regard yourself as 'A frail old thing' you are less likely to walk neatly across a narrow plank bridge. A lot of improvement in skill may be achieved simply through taking measures to improve your self-confidence and your respect for your body. Why refrain from taking part in modern dancing? Does it matter if you make a fool of yourself? Younger people are more likely to admire you for making a valiant effort. I have heard of a lady in her mid-seventies learning to swim for the first time in her life, and this is a skill that demands self-confidence.

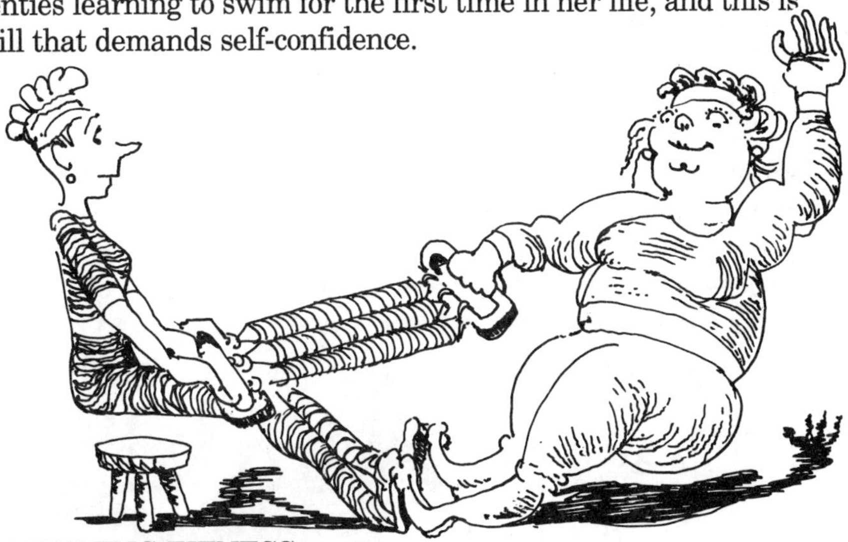

MAINTAINING FITNESS

If you can improve the fitness you never needed to lose in the first place, (unless, of course, you have gone through an extended period of illness) the same remedial measures that you employ can be incorporated into your usual life-style so that you remain fit, and the 'fitness gap', as referred to earlier, will be very small. You have to take a deliberate decision to do this, because for many years it is likely that you have had a life style that did not provide the sorts of exercise that maintain the four attributes of fitness. About the only jobs that would do this are those of the ballet dancer and the professional athlete. For the ordinary person whose job and life-style may have been principally sedentary it is therefore necessary to take active steps to maintain fitness at any age. A period of illness may have compelled you to be rather inactive for a while, but the danger is that after convalescence you will not resume the amount of exercise that was normal for you before.

You may well ask 'What sort of exercise do I need?' and that is a fair question, but the answer must depend upon your health and age – and I mean anything up to 100 – whether you still have the full use of all your limbs, and whether you have any permanent condition like a dicky heart that is relevant to exercise. In many books there is some vagueness about the nature of the exercise you should take, and how much.

Obviously a 60 year old can be expected to take more strenuous exercise than a 90 year old, but how much more? Sarah Lamb examined the whole question of exercise and the elderly in the Carnegie Third Age Inquiry and discussed it in terms of safety, effectiveness, enjoyment and cost.

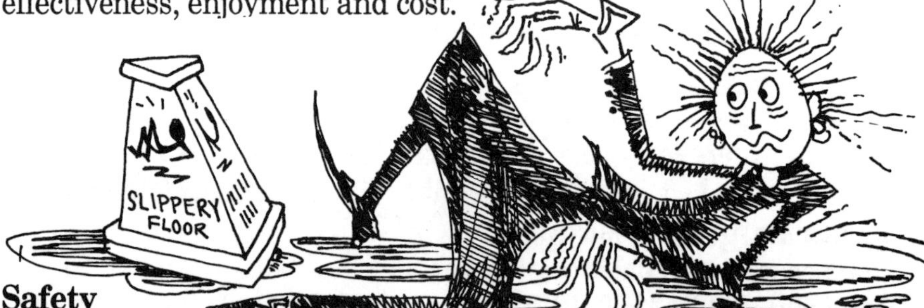

Safety

This is a serious matter for older people who, in their eagerness to keep themselves fit, may do themselves injury. But you should not be too cautious as are some people who have had heart trouble.

For instance, many older doctors used to advise people who had had a heart attack that they should regard sexual intercourse as a thing of the past because of the risk to their hearts. However, later research has shown that such caution is unnecessary. If you can walk up two flights of stairs you can certainly resume sexual intercourse after you have recovered from the attack, and a sensible doctor will tell you when you are fit for it.

Oddly enough, one study of a training programme showed that the risk of heart trouble was less for a 50 - 69 year old group than for a younger group aged 40 - 49 years old. This paradoxical finding indicates that in the older group people were more experienced in dealing with their dicky hearts, and knew when to slow down.

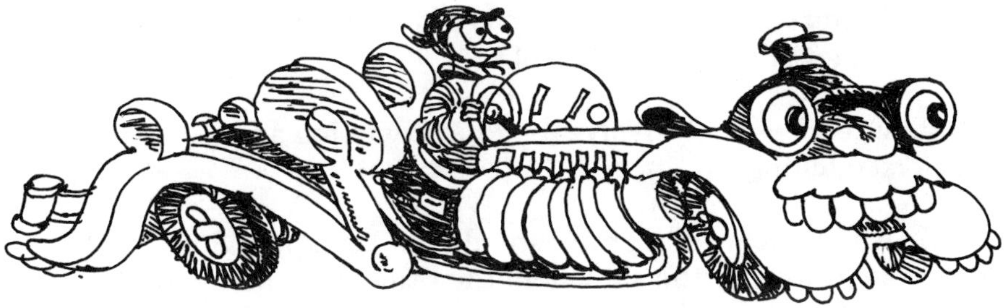

Managing an older body is like running a very old car – as the years go by you get to know its tricks and how to get the best out of it, so that you may keep it running sweetly on the road for years and years. You take it to the garage when you suspect it will need some professional attention, so with your body, you take it to the doctor's surgery for a periodic MOT and when you suspect that it needs a special check-up. By so doing you are not wasting professional time – you are saving it, for by so doing you prevent yourself from becoming an old crock who needs elaborate treatment and perhaps a hospital bed. Happily, my own GP has a hobby of tinkering with old cars and keeping them on the road.

In exercise programmes there is some danger of leaders with less than adequate qualifications. Such badly conducted programmes for older people have led, according to the Carnegie Inquiry, to a 50% toll of sprains, strains and bone injuries within the first few weeks of conditioning, and obviously you should use your common sense in avoiding what you feel is too much for you. It is you who know when to stop or slow down, not someone else. The main risks are listed below so that you can see whether any of them apply to you:

1. Clumsiness due to lack of recent practice.

2. Obesity, which puts too much strain on your joints and tendons

3. Failure to take it slowly to begin with. An experienced leader should warn you of this.

4. Exercises that involve too much twisting and stretching.

5. All members of a group should not be expected to continue for the same length of time or achieve the same standard.

6. Your own over-eagerness and a tendency to compete with others. Remember that you are there for your own individual welfare and not to win prizes.

7. A mundane but important matter – shoes without adequate heels and ankle support are a real danger.

Some researchers have tried to compile a questionnaire to assess the present status of any individual's readiness for activity training, but so far such work has been done only with young and middle-aged people. In later life you will have to go for a medical check-up if you are in doubt about your capacity for undertaking such exercise.

Effectiveness

Risks that may be involved when older people embark on an activity training programme have been described in some detail, but of course the same considerations apply in daily life if you go walking, bicycling, hill-climbing, playing golf or tennis, swimming, jogging, or undertaking any other healthful but potentially demanding exercise. There is, of course, a danger that you may take some token exercise, and imagine that you have thereby assured your health, but not really exerted yourself enough.

A walk up to the pub half a mile away every day is hardly enough to satisfy your body's needs. Whatever age you are, and in whatever condition you find yourself you should exercise until you are pleasantly tired, and that is about the best advice that can be offered. Jogging has been mentioned but can be dangerous for those with a high level of aspiration and a puritan conscience that demands that we should punish the flesh as John Knox decreed. Don't punish the flesh – learn to enjoy it. Over enthusiastic joggers, all got up in the proper kit and showing off to the younger ones, have been known to collapse by the wayside.

Enjoyment

The great impediment to taking effective exercise is boredom, and that is why exertion in a social milieu is to be recommended. To make the activity have a purpose is also an advantage. If a walk of two miles has a pub, a café, a friend's house, or other attractive target at the end of it, so much the better. Almost all U3As have 'ambling' or rambling groups, some combined with local or natural history studies, and many older people take part in walks organized by The Ramblers Association. Learn to reward yourself in the course of exercising, then you will look forward to it rather than regarding it as a dutiful chore. We all have hobbies, and if you can integrate your hobbies to include healthful exercise such as gardening, studying natural history by investigating flora and fauna in the local countryside, and other purposeful trips on foot or bicycle, so much the better.

Cost

Fitness classes that have a trained leader obviously cost money, and local authorities tend to be not over-generous in making facilities available, but nowadays many self-help organizations for older people are springing up; I would make special mention of the University of the Third Age which, despite sounding rather academic, organizes all sorts of active recreational pursuits such as swimming, 'Third Age dance', Yoga, T'ai Chi Chuan, tennis, badminton, table tennis, weight training and rambling. Because these are organized specifically for oldies there is no problem of competing with younger people who may resent the presence of slow, clumsy elders. As for cost, it is normal for members who have some relevant talents (e.g. as swimming instructors) to give their services free, and the fees are kept to a minimum, some hard-up OAPs being admitted free in special cases.

There are local Universities of the Third Age all over the country almost everyone of which has a walking group, and the address of the central office is given in Appendix A.

SEVEN OLD WIVES' TALES

Let's be frank; many of us oldies know very well that we ought to take more exercise for the sake of our health but we just can't be bothered. Are you in this category? When we want to wriggle out of a duty, even if it's only a duty to ourselves, it is handy to have a few ready excuses, and it is of interest to study the excuses that people have given for their inactivity. Some people make use of old wives' tales as excuses, and they may even believe in them.

In one social survey of older people some remarkable excuses were given for inactivity, even blaming the Almighty ('It's God's will').

Not all inactive older people give excuses: an old friend of mine drank like a fish and smoked like a chimney, and seldom ventured beyond his own garden. He was very poor and denied himself food in order to spend money on beer and cigarettes, saying quite cheerfully 'If I choose to smoke myself to death that's my business.' He lived to a surprisingly late age with a horrible smoker's cough, but he was a merry old man to the end and died of an ailment quite unrelated to his lungs or heart. If the ideal of a (possibly) short, lazy and perhaps boozy life is yours, good luck to you and you need make no excuses to anyone. However, many of the excuses that inactive people make stem from mistaken beliefs and attitudes, and if they were not so misinformed they would be able to make more rational choices. Here are seven old wives' tales about ageing, ideas that have long been discredited, but still linger on and lead to sad excuses for self-neglect. Are you influenced by any of them?

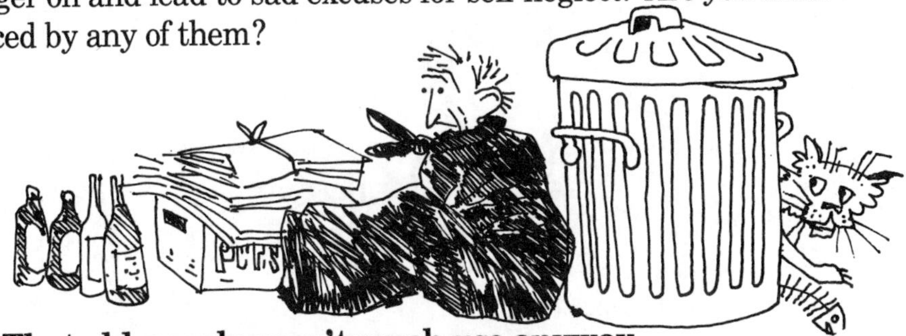

1. **That old people aren't much use anyway**

Some people tend to lose their self-esteem, and hence stop caring for themselves as they used to when they were younger when they felt that they were valuable members of society. Unfortunately, the negative beliefs about ageing and old people that were common in their younger years have affected their own image, and they need to have their self-respect restored before they will begin to listen to any advice about looking after their health.

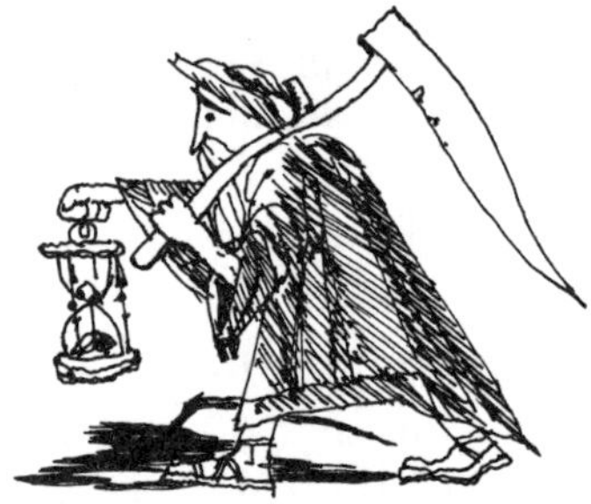

2. **That after sixty death is imminent**

One of the sad excuses that are occasionally given can be expressed as 'Well, I haven't got much longer to live anyway, so why bother?' This comes from older people who haven't woken up to the fact that nowadays we may expect to live to a rather greater age than formerly, and it's better to live on healthily, and hence happily, than as an old crock.

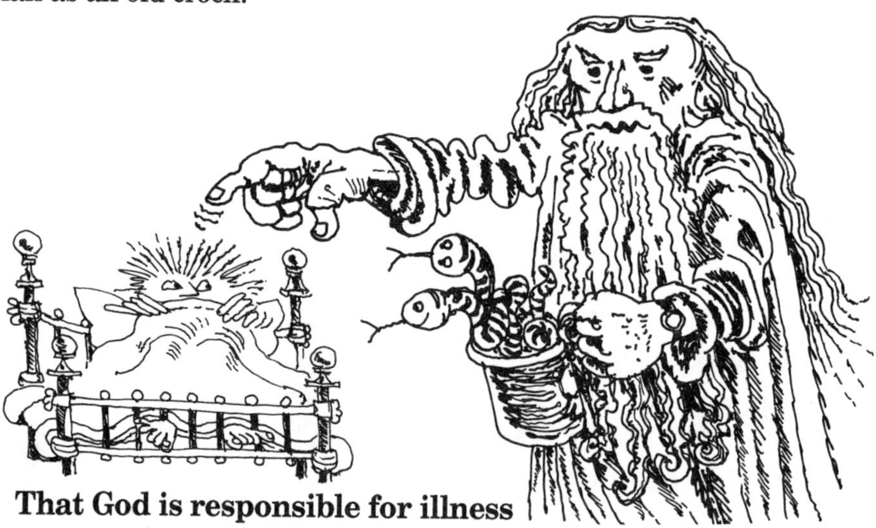

3. **That God is responsible for illness**

This extraordinary belief is sometimes held by religious people of a number of different faiths. They see disease and disability as being caused by God who allows it to afflict some people and not others. *The Book of Job* is of course an expression of this belief. They say as they commute from bed to armchair and back again, wheezing as they climb the stairs, 'It's the will of God'.

I know of a lady who became, not an atheist, but bitterly anti-God for the last five years of her life when she was practically bed-ridden. She had lived a very moral and religious life, and regarded it as grossly unfair that she had to spend the last part of it in such misery. Presumably, according to this belief, the thoroughly wicked sinners who start in later life to take plenty of healthful exercise, cut down on the booze, stop smoking, and carefully consider what they eat, are additionally wicked because they are flying in the face of the Almighty who intends them to be ill.

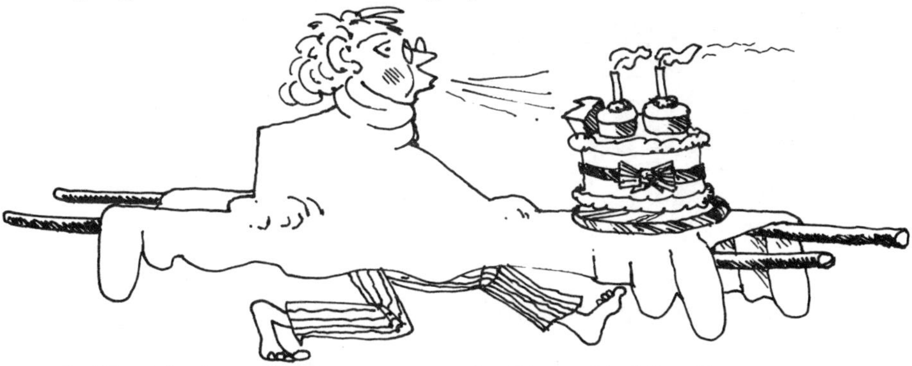

4. **That being old is some sort of inevitable disease**

This false belief is very common, and unfortunately it has been fostered by a minority of doctors, now happily small. Quite a number of people believe that their various aches and pains, their shortness of breath, and other disabilities are the natural result of being old. The doctor who says, 'Well, what can you expect at your age anyway?' is fostering this myth.

There is the tale of a man aged 101 who went to his doctor complaining of stiffness in his right knee, and the doctor laughed and said 'Look, that knee of yours is 101 years old, so what can you expect?' The old man replied 'Well, my left knee is also 101 years old and it's all right, so what are you going to do about it?' Those who believe in this old wives' tale about the equivalence of age and disability see no reason to seek professional help for their various ailments.

Their reaction can be summed up as, 'Well, it's my age isn't it?' They have difficulty in accepting the idea that they can significantly reduce their ailments and regain a lot of their fitness by seeking professional advice and taking proper exercise.

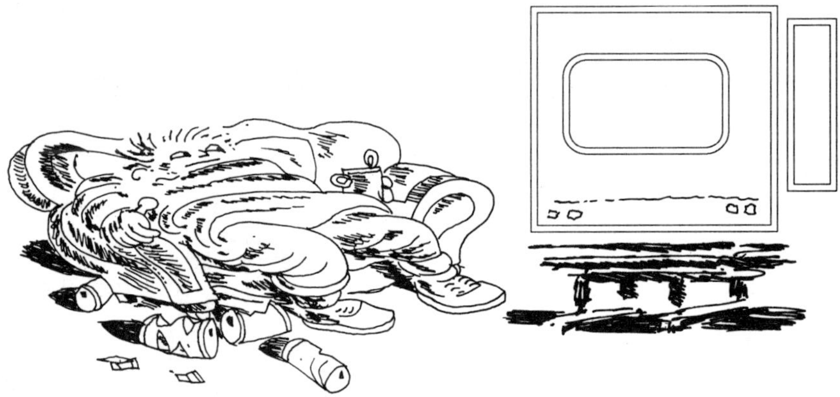

5. **That you can wear your body out by exercise**

Some people, as they slump in front of the TV screen, excuse their inactivity by saying 'I don't want to wear my body out'. While it is true that a life of gross over-work is likely to be a short one, especially when accompanied by a poor diet as in the abuse of slaves, we have evolved from our hunter-gatherer ancestors to sustain a lot more physical work that we normally accomplish, except, perhaps in primitive farming communities. The curious idea that we are endowed with a certain quantity of work-potential to last our lives, and that it may be used up, goes by the name of 'entropy', a concept that is falsely derived from physics.

The same word used to be applied also to sexual energy – the false belief that if a person was very active sexually in their youth they would have little sexual capacity in later life. In fact in both, as applied to work and sex, the exact contrary is true; the more you use a capacity the better it is preserved.

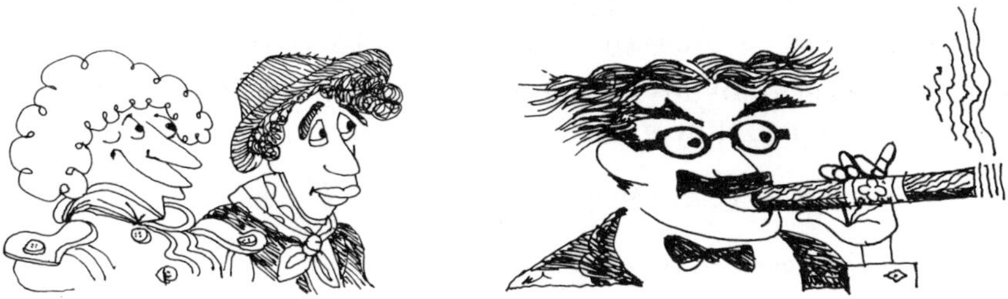

6. **That now you're old, who would look at you anyway?**

The epitome of self-denigration is expressed in Groucho Marx's reply when he was asked why he had never joined any club: 'Why should I want to join a club that would have me as a member?'

It must be admitted that one reason for keeping our general looks is that we want to look attractive to other people – especially the opposite sex. This may be condemned as vanity by John Knox – but why not admit it? Most people are quite frank about it when they are young, but there is a myth that over a certain age we look so awful anyway that we might as well give up and be content with sagging, over-fat bellies and hunched shoulders. This is part of the negative stereotype of the elderly that has been challenged by the generation who have more recently entered the Third Age.

It is well established now that many people in later life who become single for one reason or another do form new partnerships, and perhaps to their great surprise, fall in love and find other people falling in love with them. But pair-bonding apart, you want your friends and age-mates around you to look pleasant, and even in spite of wrinkles, we can look quite attractive if we are healthy, so it is up to us to keep ourselves in good shape.

I have not mentioned it so far, but not only does physical exercise improve our bodily wellbeing but it improves our mental state as well. If you want to be cheerful and lighthearted, do not shun looking in the mirror; you may not be the raving beauty or the handsome masher that you used to be, but you can still make the best of yourself. Look in the mirror, a full-length mirror, and study how you can present yourself to the world. As for your face, remember John Donne's lines:

No spring, nor summer beauty hath such grace,

As I have seen in one autumnal face.

Why should not that apply to your autumnal face?

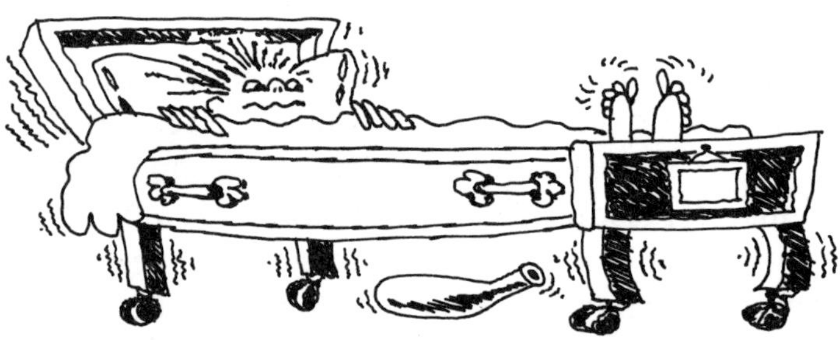

7. That when you are ill you should stay in bed until you are better

In 1947 a pioneering doctor, Richard Asher, published an amusing article in the *British Medical Journal* entitled 'The dangers of going to bed'. At that time it was common for patients to be kept in bed for inordinately long periods (six week bed-rest for an attack of coronary thrombosis!). Asher attacked this practice pointing out that such enforced rest was entirely unnecessary, and actually retarded recovery from many disorders. He quoted the hymn:

Teach me to live that I may dread

The grave as little as my bed

and suggested that doctors should sing his amended version:

Teach us to live that we may dread

Unnecessary time in bed.

Get people up that we may save

Our patients from an early grave.

Medicine is a very conservative profession, and it was a long time before the advice of pioneers such as Richard Asher took effect. When I had my first coronary attack in 1961 I came under the care of quite an old consultant, and he condemned me to a bed-rest so complete that I was forbidden even to feed myself. At mealtimes a junior nurse had to stand by me and spoon food into my mouth, a slow and tedious process. Once she was doing this and gossiping to another nurse over her shoulder; her inattentiveness resulted in a spoonful being ladled into my ear instead of my mouth. I recovered from the heart attack quite quickly, but it was a long while before I recovered from the extended bed-rest.

When I had my next coronary attack 15 years later (I have had three as I have a typically A Type personality – I will discuss the significance of this anon) I was not moved to hospital, and the doctor, a young and progressive chap, just told me to get up when I felt better, and to take it easy for a bit.

Asher pointed out that patients in hospital were kept in bed for long periods not for any medical reason, but because it made the wards so much tidier, with everyone stacked away like plates in a dish-rack, and the practice greatly appealed to ward sisters. According to Dr Alex Comfort:

Older people in Britain are spared the excesses of the American nursing-home racket; there fit people are kept in bed because the owners get higher subventions for the bedridden. Here they may be kept unnecessarily in bed because it's tidier like that . . . It is an old idea that the best thing for any illness is rest in bed. In older people bed rest can be a killer. There are obvious conditions where one must stay in bed – fevers and severe colds are two of them – but make it a rule never to stay in bed longer than two days, after the age of sixty-five, without checking with the doctor. Apart from lung and blood-clotting problems, the muscles waste and the bones decalcify much faster in the old than the young, and in the very old a few days' confinement to bed can make them really weak. When bed rest is necessary, there are ways of avoiding this, but they need expert supervision.

The trouble is that the people who are now old grew up in an age when bed-rest in the home was considered the appropriate remedy for almost every ill, and because of this old wives' tale they are apt to do themselves injury by resorting to bed all too easily. One specialist in medicine for the elderly looks to the future with hope for he says that although those who are now old cling to this mistaken idea, those who will be old in the next century were not so conditioned in their attitudes by the past, and he adds a dig at some of his colleagues:

> They will, hopefully, be advised by professionals who are more aware of the benefits of exercise than today's professionals . . . It is probable therefore that exercise promotion will play a much more prominent part in the delivery of health and social services in future than it does today.

But you may say that, illness apart, you enjoy your bed and look upon lounging there, sometimes until very late in the morning, as a positive pleasure. Sure, if it is a pleasure by all means enjoy it, and your pleasure may be enhanced by a breakfast tray, a book, or a pleasant companion. In the latter case your rest may be mixed with some very pleasant and healthful exercise. The enjoyment of your bed is not at all incompatible with a proper amount of exercise when you are up and about, for remember that the message of this book is 'A little of what you fancy does you good'.

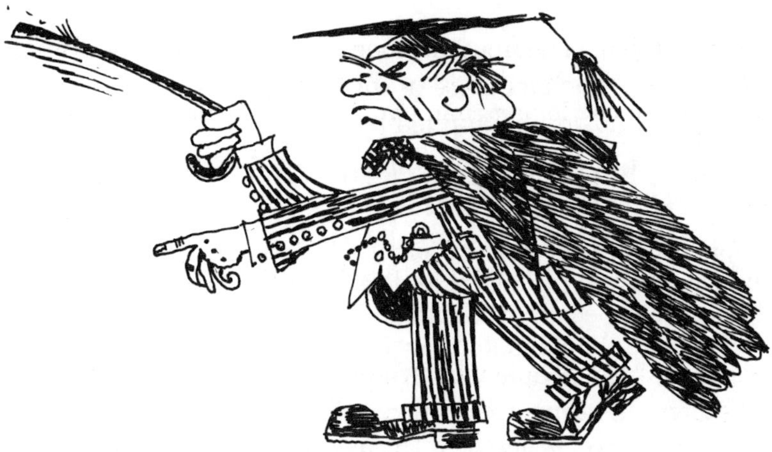

ARE WE OLDIES ENTIRELY TO BLAME?

I may have given the impression in this chapter that all the people in the Third Age are lazily ignoring the good advice about taking proper exercise that the health-professionals as a body are trying to present to them. You may resent such a presentation, and say that it is certainly not true of you. This picture would indeed be false, and the position is more complex than that. A number of doctors and other health professionals have still to learn all that modern research can teach about health in later life, and to implement it in their practice.

When Jean McHeath carried out a survey of beliefs and attitudes among thirdagers and among health-professionals, she discovered some surprising facts about people's understanding of health issues and the importance of exercise in maintaining fitness. She found that 82% of her sample of elderly people believed that exercise was 'what is wanted and needed', and that it was 'important, necessary and good', whereas only 62% of the health-professionals were positive about this. As many as 14% of the latter engaged in rehabilitative work with older people said that talking to them about exercise was unimportant and a waste of time, but the elderly people thought that professionals should go to the trouble of explaining about the benefits of exercise.

There is always a gap of quite a number of years before the findings of research, such as those of the Carnegie Inquiry, become generally known and applied by the public. I should like to end this chapter by quoting an important expert in the health of thirdagers, Dr Muir Gray:

Elderly people do not exist in isolation. They exist in society, being influenced by, and influencing, other groups. They cannot, and should not, be expected to change in isolation, and education for health in old age should not simply be directed at people who are growing old or who are old; everybody, including highly trained professionals, require education to help them cope with the major challenge that is posed by the ageing of our population.'

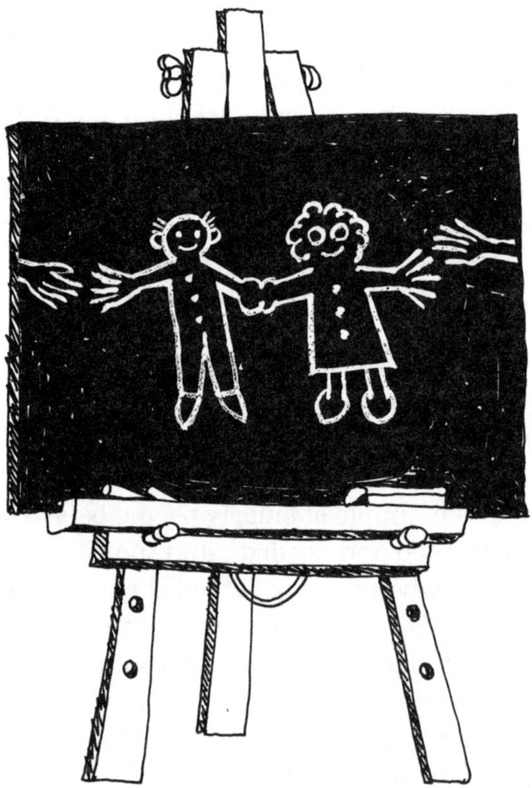

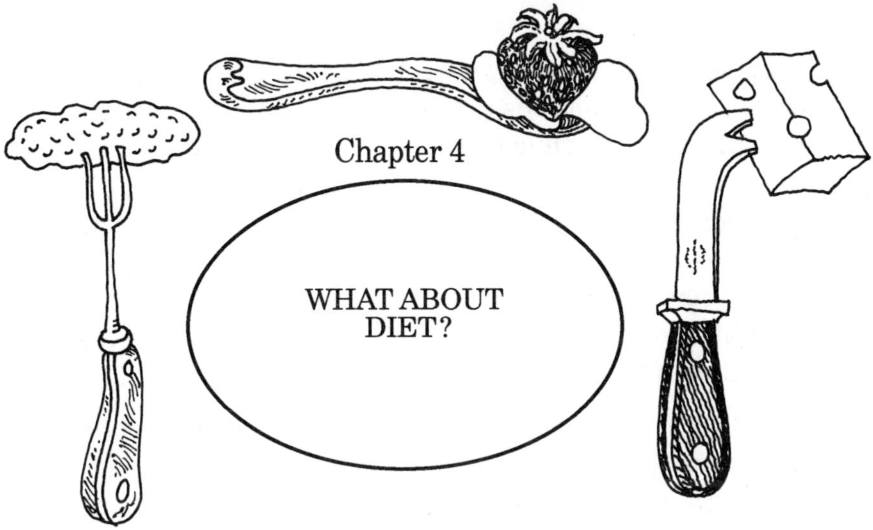

Chapter 4

WHAT ABOUT DIET?

You may well ask, 'Do I need a special diet in later life?', and the answer is unquestionably, 'No, and don't let anyone fool you that you do; but you've got to use your head about some important matters if you are to remain healthy.'

As you get older there is a slowing down of the chemical processes in the body that concern the burning and utilization of food. This process is known as the 'basal metabolic rate', and it varies very much from individual to individual. It is perfectly natural that although you may take adequate exercise appropriate to your age, you are not as active as you used to be, therefore you don't need to eat as much.

Healthy people eat a good mixed diet, and most people in the western world thrive on it, as the steadily falling rate of mortality in the population has shown. However, it is as well to note that in some parts of the UK still more improvement is needed; in some regions far too much fat and sugar is eaten, with inevitable consequences of ill-health, as will be discussed later.

It is important to preserve a mixed diet (for reasons I shall discuss later) and the principle of 'a little of what you fancy does you good' is upheld by all modern nutritionists. It is true that in special cases some populations can remain healthy on a remarkably limited range of staple foods, but only when they get the balance right; when the balance is not right, they die out. In the early nineteenth century a lot of the Irish peasant population lived almost exclusively on potatoes, milk and butter, but the potato is a truly remarkable vegetable, and they must have eaten huge quantities of them, and various little extras that are easily available to country people.

Any discussion of diet is bedevilled by considerations that have nothing to do with food values. You are urged not to eat this or that for ethical reasons which I do not intend to debate here but, in my opinion, they have nothing to do with nutrition. Second, you are urged to eat this or that because food manufacturers aim to make money out of you, and hence they spend millions on advertising certain foodstuffs, but again, the commercial interests of the manufacturers are an issue separate from the nutritional value of their products.

THE CONSTITUENTS OF FOOD

Your diet consists of three classes of food: protein, carbohydrate and fat. As food occurs in nature it also includes tiny quantities of vitamins and minerals, and these are essential for a healthy diet. However we get our food, it naturally includes a lot of plant fibre and the indigestible part of meat. All this, which is known as 'roughage' is necessary for the gut to be bulked out as it extracts the nourishment from the food.

Protein

Protein in greater or lesser quantities is present in almost all kinds of foodstuffs, with the exception of those that are pure fat (butter, cooking oil) and sugar and alcohol. Although there is protein in foods as different as apples and fish, some foods are specially rich in protein such as meat and cheese, and that is why you follow your tastes and include such protein-rich foods in 'solid' meals.

Carbohydrates

You consume most of your carbohydrate in the form of starch and sugar – in bread, potatoes, rice, pasta etc. Sugar is added in food preparation, or direct from the sugar bowl, partly because you like the taste of it, and you know by experience that it gives you immediate energy.

Some Cambridge scientists did an experiment investigating how old, as compared with young, people reacted to sugar. They invited two groups of people, one old and one young, to come for an experiment in the morning not having eaten breakfast that day. They were all given a drink of a slightly sweet liquid: half the drinks were sweetened with saccharine (which has no food value) and half with glucose, a form of sugar that is not very sweet so you can take a lot of it without noticing. They were then given tests of learning and memory.

It made no difference to the performance of the younger group whether they had had the glucose drink, but the half of the older group who had drunk the sugared drink performed better. That this was due to the difference in the level of their blood-sugar was confirmed by testing samples of their blood. It is apparent, therefore, that when you are older you need to top up your blood sugar in the mornings, and it is therefore inadvisable to skip breakfast if you want to perform at your best but you don't need to add sugar from the sugar bowl at breakfast, since the starch in your toast or cornflakes is soon converted to sugar.

Fat

You need fat in some form or other, and you generally get it as margarine, butter, cooking oil or bacon fat. Plenty of other natural foods such as nuts, fish and olives contain fats, saturated and unsaturated. The former class, which occurs principally in meat and dairy products, tends to produce an excess of cholesterol in the blood, and older people should therefore consciously limit their use of it because of the danger of heart trouble and strokes.

There is another reason why you may have to be careful about eating too much fatty food, because it has a very high food value, and if you have a tendency to obesity in later life, you have to watch it!

The question of fat people will be dealt with later; there is no harm in being rather chubby, the danger lies in becoming over-fat.

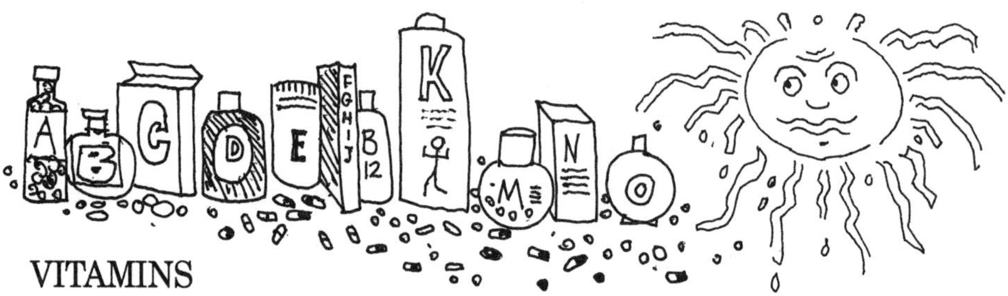

VITAMINS

Vitamins are chemicals that occur in very tiny amounts in most foodstuffs, and if you eat a normal mixed diet, as most people do in the western world, you get all the vitamins you need and a little more. The diseases of vitamin deficiency – notably scurvy, beriberi, and pellagra – which used to affect some of our malnourished ancestors, and still affect some people in the third world, are virtually unknown in modern Europe because most of us eat a mixed diet. Nevertheless, vitamins are a rich source of profit for those quacks who seek to bamboozle the public by misleading them about the necessity for extra vitamins and other food supplements that they don't really need.

Vitamin C

You may have read on some cartons of the juice of fruits that already contain plenty of vitamin C the manufacturers' statement 'With added vitamin C.' Do you know what happens when you have enough vitamin C in your body already, as most of us have, and you drink such a juice? Next time you visit the lavatory the extra vitamin that the manufacturers have added in order to boast about it (and increase the price) goes down the drain unaltered.

Some old people live in circumstances that mean they get rather less than the full amount of vitamin C which is good for them. Vitamin C, which occurs principally in fruits and vegetables, is the vitamin that is rather easily destroyed by too much cooking, by the prolonged storage of cooked food, and by keeping food hot for too long. Some thirdagers may be getting insufficient Vitamin C if:

(a) they are very hard up because of their inadequate pensions;

(b) having lived frugally during the years of the war and rationing, they are apt to hoard left-overs and heat them up;

(c) they have to depend on 'meals on wheels'.

If the latter service is being administered properly then they should receive freshly-cooked hot meals that have not been stored too long in the process of transport and delivery. But what if the recipient does not eat the meal immediately, and keeps it until the next day and reheats it ? It should be made clear that such meals are to be eaten straight away or the vitamin value may be seriously depleted. No great harm will come to them if they do not follow this rule on every occasion, but if they neglect it month after month they are not getting a proper diet, as well as putting themselves at risk of food-poisoning, which will be discussed later.

If you eat a truly mixed diet including fresh fruit and vegetables, sources rich in protein such as meat, fish, cheese, eggs, beans, milk, and carbohydrates in bread, potatoes, pasta, etc., plus some but not too much of fatty foods, you do not need to worry about your vitamin intake. Do not be conned into buying the various vitamin pills that unscrupulous manufacturers advertise in such glowing terms. They tend to be wary of claiming that 'Scientists have shown that vitamin Q will restore the colour of your hair, remove wrinkles from your skin and improve your sexual potency' because the Advertising Standards Authority would prosecute them for telling such thumping great lies, but their ploy is to state that some people suggest such wonders can be derived from vitamin Q, so why not give it a try?

There are some abnormal conditions that occur in later life that call for extra vitamins in the diet but it is best to seek the advice of your doctor who will prescribe what you may need to take and any adjustments to your diet that are necessary. Don't try self-medication until you rattle like a pill-box. It is possible to injure your health by over-dosing with vitamins, as I shall explain later.

Vitamin A

This is a fat-soluble vitamin and hence you get it in ample quantities in dairy products, margarine (where it is added in the manufacturing process), oily fish like herrings, and, oddly enough, you can get it by eating carrots. A curious tale derives from the latter fact: during the war there was propaganda stating that fighter-pilots were given carrots to eat because it improves night-vision. So it does, but it would be difficult to find many people in the population whose night-vision was defective because they lacked enough vitamin A!

The real reason for this quaint lie was that the government wished to mislead the enemy and conceal the fact that now the fighter-pilots had got a form of radar which assisted their perception of enemy planes.

You store vitamin A in your liver, and you are probably carrying about a year's supply of it, so it does not matter if you don't eat another carrot or herring for months as far as your vitamin A supply is concerned. Because carnivorous animals that eat a lot of oily prey are at the top of the food chain, they accumulate large quantities of vitamin A in their livers, and the polar bear has a liver so rich in this vitamin that it is dangerous to eat it. Eskimos learnt this over centuries of trial and error, so when they kill such a bear they will not eat the liver and hide it from their dogs.

Vitamin B group

More than half a dozen vitamins are classed in this group, and they are very common in a lot of foodstuffs, principally in wholemeal bread, various cereals, meat, liver, and peanuts. The deficiency diseases of beri-beri and pellagra, are due to shortages of vitamins in this group, and used to occur in peasant populations. Some cornflake packages bear the statement 'With added vitamin B', but needless to say this additive is quite unnecessary unless you are a maize-eating peasant living on an impoverished diet.

Vitamin D

Like vitamin A this is an oil-soluble vitamin, and the two vitamins often occur together. Vitamin D is important for children as it is necessary for the building up of bones, and that is why children were given cod-liver oil during the war, as deficiency of it leads to rickets. Because this vitamin is also important for pregnant women who are building up the skeletons of their babies they may need extra vitamin D. As young and middle-aged adults already have their skeletons formed they don't have to worry about vitamin D, but there is a certain condition in later life known as osteomalacia where the proper structure of the bones is not maintained and therefore, under medical supervision, they need to adjust their diet by eating foods that are rich in the vitamin, and perhaps take supplements.

Vitamin D is manufactured in your body when the skin is exposed to sunlight, and that is why children who live in conditions where they get little sunlight may be liable to rickets unless they get a diet rich in vitamin D. Similarly the children and some old people in immigrant communities who come from sunny lands may be at risk if they stick to ethnic diets that were appropriate in their sun-drenched homelands but which lack the normal amount of vitamin D that occurs in the diets of the people of northern Europe.

Vitamin D in gross excess can also be dangerous to health, as is illustrated by the following clinical case: a lady aged 79 was brought to a hospital by her daughter because she appeared to be 'senile'. She refused practically all food and had given up talking to anyone. The tests at the hospital showed no abnormal features in her physiology, except a raised level of calcium in her blood.

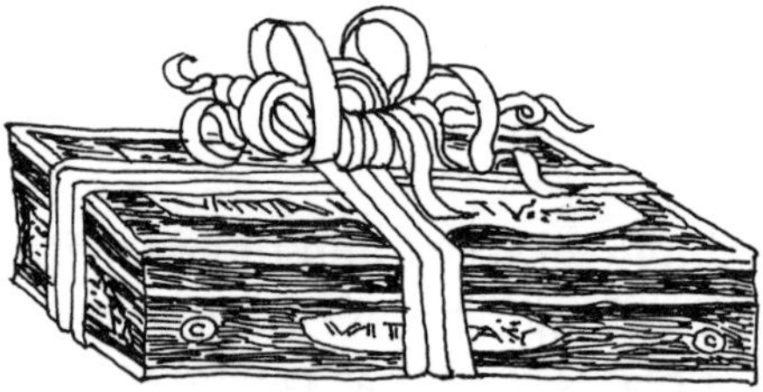

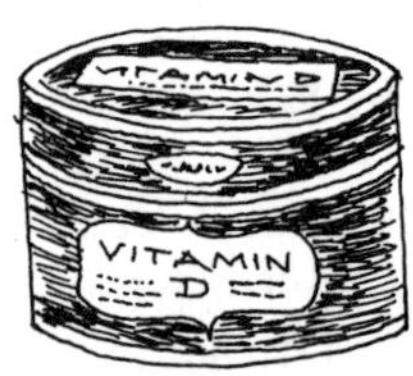

During her stay in hospital this lady returned to normal, eating, talking to other people and reading, and so the mysterious illness appeared to have terminated and she was discharged. At the final interview with the doctors her daughter mentioned her mother's 'medicine'. Further inquiry revealed that she had been taking vitamin pills; these were pills containing vitamin D, and the manufacturers, hoping to increase their sales, had coated them with chocolate. As this lady was very fond of chocolate she had begun to consume more and more of them and eventually ended up with consuming 150,000 units of vitamin D a day, thus poisoning herself and going into a state that resembled dementia. Be warned – some vitamin pills can seriously damage your health if you grossly exceed the maximum daily dose.

It must be noted that oily fish, although an excellent food for most people and a source of vitamin D, has its risks for some older people. Those who have a tendency to develop gout in later life should be warned that oily fish is one of the foods which may precipitate an attack, so go easy on the herring, mackerel, and fish-roe if you have this disability. All doctors are not aware of this apparently, for once when I went to a doctor with a gouty foot she prescribed a drug and added that perhaps I should keep off tomatoes!

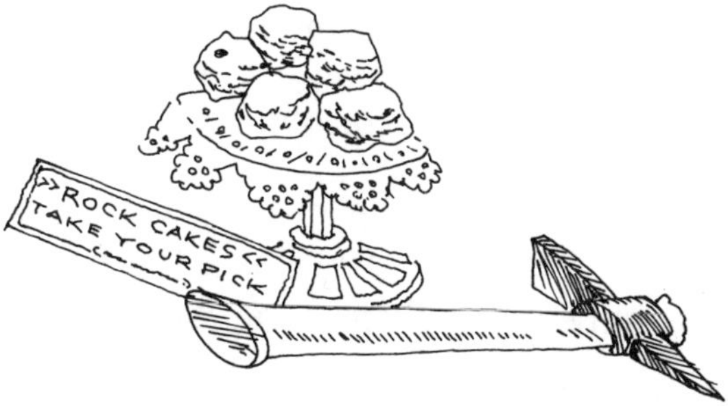

MINERALS

Certain minerals are necessary for health, and they occur in so many foods that you do not need to bother about them provided you have a good mixed diet. It is only in very special circumstances that a diet is deficient in all the necessary minerals: for instance, in parts of Derbyshire the drinking water is so deficient in iodine that the natives used to develop 'Derbyshire neck', that is a swelling of the thyroid gland (goitre), and gross absence of iodine from the diet, as used to occur in some parts of Peru, results in the physical stunting of children and a form of mental deficiency known as cretinism.

Calcium

Calcium is an essential mineral in food, and it is necessary for children to get an adequate supply of it as it goes to build up the skeleton; this is one of the reasons why all schoolchildren used to be supplied with free milk, a measure which was introduced in wartime. Unfortunately, the bones of people late in life which may become thin and soft cannot be benefited however much calcium-rich food is in their diet. As mentioned above, osteomalacia, the condition of softening of the bones, may be treated with vitamin D; the condition is not normally due to lack of calcium in the diet but the inability to utilize it.

Osteoporosis, the condition in which the bones become brittle and may occur much earlier in life, cannot be treated by adding extra calcium to the diet, so don't be fooled by quack advertisements. This latter condition is related to the balance of hormones, particularly after the menopause. However, in the long term an adequate mixed diet containing the many sources of calcium will help to maintain a robust skeleton in later life.

Another factor that is responsible for the retention of calcium is exercise, for, as was mentioned previously, those who spend too many days lying in bed steadily lose the calcium from their bones.

Salt

Common table salt, which is almost entirely composed of sodium chloride, is taken for granted and used a great deal in cooking to improve the flavour of food. It is a necessary mineral in food, and in parts of the world where it does not occur naturally in the soil in sufficient quantities it becomes a valuable item of commerce.

It provides a good example of a little of what you fancy doing you good, for salt-deprived humans and animals avidly seek it, guided by their taste and (in animals) smell. Most people add salt to many kinds of food at the table, and some develop a fondness for it far beyond their need for it.

As a salty diet raises the blood-pressure, there is a danger of hypertensive older people eating too much. Eating salt because you fancy it is one thing, but you should beware of sprinkling your food out of habit; it is a bad habit especially for older people.

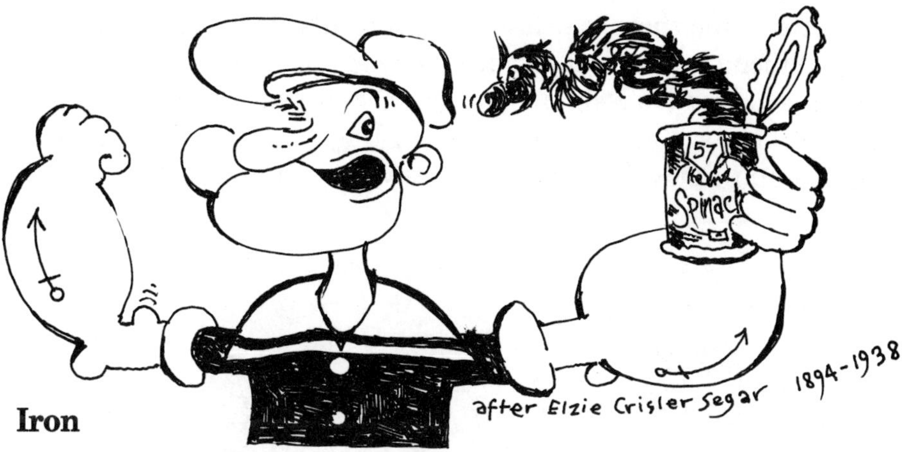

Iron

This is one of the few minerals that may be deficient in an ordinary diet, as even when it is abundantly present in a food, it may not be in a form that is easily absorbed. A classic case is Popeye's spinach. This cartoon character is depicted as reaching for a can of spinach whenever he is in a tight corner and needing extra strength, the common-sense connection being made, iron = strength.

Popeye has doubtless been invoked by many mothers anxious that their children should eat up their spinach. Although this vegetable does indeed contain plenty of iron, as do many other plants, it is unfortunately in a form not easily absorbed in the human gut.

Sources rich in iron in a form that we can absorb are: meat – especcially liver; any foodstuff containing blood, such as black pudding; grapes – raisins, currants and sultanas; cocoa powder; black treacle, a cheap spread that used to be popular in poor households.

Those who have difficulty in absorbing iron, or who have a diet deficient in it as do some vegetarians who do not plan their diet carefully, may develop anaemia. Although anaemia is not common nowadays, older people suffer from it more than young. Those who are eking out their lives on inadequate pensions tend to eat very little meat, and those who have ill-fitting false teeth tend to find meat difficult to chew. If you are prone to anaemia, not only should you include foods rich in iron in your diet, but you should also eat plenty of green vegetables, for they contain a vitamin of the B group, folic acid, which enables you to absorb iron.

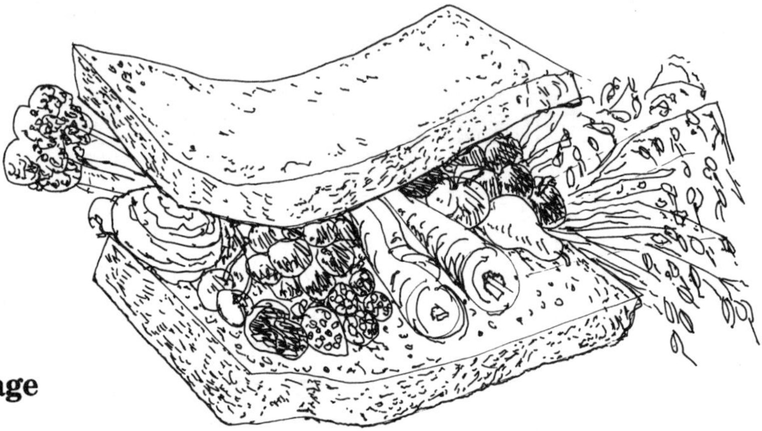

Roughage

This is composed of substances that have no nutritional value but are essential in the digestive process to bulk out the contents of the intestines so that they may be smoothly passed along. A common complaint of older people is that they suffer from constipation, and this is most often due to the fact that they do not eat enough roughage.

You should never, never depend upon swallowing laxatives unless they are prescribed by your doctor – the laxative habit can be most dangerous. Roughage is mainly supplied by the fibres of vegetables and fruit, and the bran in wholemeal bread. During the earlier part of this century patent medicine firms did a roaring trade by selling laxatives which were widely advertised. Fashions in patent medicine advertising have changed, but some older people may still be affected by their memories of Mr Kruschen and his salts.

VEGETARIANISM

A perfectly healthy vegetarian diet involves more careful planning than an ordinary diet that includes meat, and this is especially important in northern countries. In sun-drenched parts of the world such as India they do not need to be so concerned with the fat soluble vitamins that are manufactured in the skin in sunlight, and they have developed their own traditional vegetarian diets.

There are roughly three sorts of vegetarians: those who just abstain from meat, referred to as the 'ovo-lacto-vegetarians' (they eat eggs and dairy produce), the lacto-vegetarians (who eat dairy produce but not eggs), and the vegans who rigidly exclude from their diet all animal products even honey. The latter, the vegans, will not eat anything that exploits the animal world, for instance, by eating honey we rob the bees of the products of their labour.

Apart from those who just do not like meat, and are revolted by it, vegetarians follow the ethical argument that the human species has no moral right to kill or exploit other animal species. There is also the ethical argument that it is wrong to devote a large acreage of land to the raising of cattle and sheep, since that acreage, if used to produce crops of vegetables and corn, could yield a far greater quantity of food to feed the hungry world. These are perfectly valid points of view but they are irrelevant to the question of whether a vegetarian or a meat-eating diet is the healthier.

Those who hold strong opinions based on ethical convictions are apt to argue that a vegetarian regime is the healthier diet, but this cannot be factually proved, one way or the other. It is difficult indeed to define what a 'vegetarian' diet should consist of; should the vegetarian drink milk, as many do, (although dairy farming involves the slaughter of calves)? Most vegetarians, except the strict vegans, do consume animal products as described above, and many disagree about what should be included. The more strictly vegetarian a diet is the more complex it becomes, for it is difficult to include all the components necessary for health if they are entirely of vegetable origin.

An interesting aspect of the vegan diet is that as it excludes all animal products it is totally deficient in vitamin B12, as this vitamin does not occur in plants except for a few seaweeds. This vitamin is essential for health, although we need only a tiny amount of it

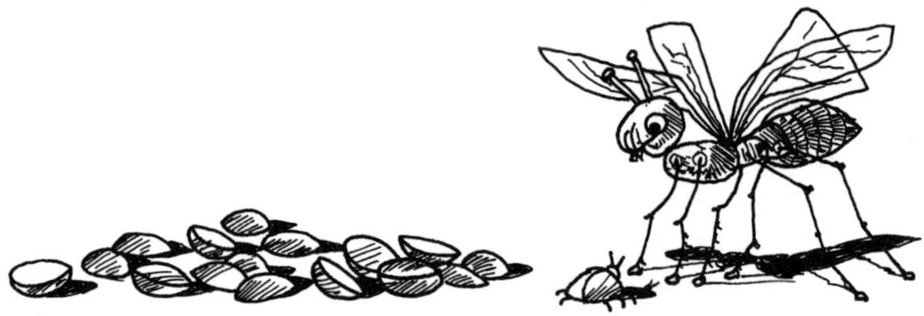

When vegans came to live in Britain as immigrants, usually from India, a few of them, notably the older people, began to suffer from a form of anaemia that occurs when people are deprived of vitamin B12. It is most likely that in India they were getting the vitamin by the contamination of their foodstuffs by bacteria and insect life, so they were in fact consuming an animal product without knowing it, but when they came to live in Britain they were deprived of it. To remedy this the vegan communities began to prepare the vitamin using bacteria and yeasts, and adding the product to their meals.

THOSE MIRACULOUS FOODS AND FOOD ADDITIVES

Many of the products sold in the so-called 'Health' shops rely more on faith than scientific evidence for the claims that are made about their nutritive values, says Magnus Pyke, an eminent British nutritional scientist:

Besides harmless, if costly, 'health foods', however, many so-called 'health food' shops also sell 'nonsense' articles that purport to cure this disease or prevent that – tablets and pills, nostrums and powders, seaweed extracts and exotic apple concentrates. The claims put forward for many of these are quite groundless. Not only do they cost money, and not only do they not fulfil the promises made on their behalf, but they also mislead people about the real nature of nutritional science, especially what it can do for health and what it cannot. There is no food which will fill you with ebullient health whenever you are feeling gloomy.

Older people are, of course, special targets for those who advertise 'health' foods and miraculous food additives, and there are several reasons for this targeting:

1. Older people suffer from minor ailments more frequently and are seeking remedies for less than perfect health.

2. Taste and smell sometimes alter in later life and people wonder whether something is wrong with their normal diet – has it been irradiated, poisoned with pesticides, rendered 'unnatural'.

3. A few older men believe in the myth that their failing sexual potency can be restored by special food additives.

4. A justifiable fear of obesity affects some older people if they become 'couch potatoes' and they seek an easy remedy through eating special foods and food additives.

5. Many advertisers assume that oldies are a bit weak in the head, and are therefore a lucrative market.

I resent the assumption that older people are necessarily weak in the head; their manifest gullibility in buying valueless food additives sold by post, in 'health' shops, and more recently in respectable chemists, is due, in my opinion, to the fact that they grew up in an age before the advertisers' art of deception had developed to its modern pitch of sophistication. Although we have always known that advertisers greatly exaggerate the merits of the products they offer, it is a comparatively new phenomenon to sell utterly worthless goods by the sheer power of clever advertising. It used to be done by cheap-jacks in market places imposing on ignorant people, but nowadays it is done by glossy magazines with apparently respectable credentials.

The exploitation of the elderly is even more advanced in the USA and Professor Terence Kuske of the Georgia Institute of Human Nutrition says much the same as Magnus Pyke:

> Aging individuals . . . begin to note aches and pains where they never occurred before. Their vigour and their ability to withstand exercise begins to decline. With decreased activity, and oftentimes increased affluence, caloric usage declines while caloric intake stays the same or increases. The resultant obesity leads to a continuing search for the "easy way out" in the form of new and glamorous diets that are published in popular magazines and are found lining the shelves of bookstores.

Professor Kuske goes on to describe a number of popular fad diets to give some guidance as to what books and magazines are merely a rip-off, and what are scientifically valid. He suggests that you should avoid books that start with testimonials of individuals as they are generally not scientific, and look at the academic credentials of the authors. He adds, 'These few simple recommendations may help to avoid being bilked by the practitioners of the food quackery business'.

CAN ANY DIET INCREASE YOUR LIFE-SPAN?

The search for an elixir to increase longevity has a very long history, and when experimental scientists found that they could indeed increase the life-span of rats it seemed that one day they might be able to increase the longevity of human beings. Briefly, it was found that by restricting the amount of food that they fed to rats, either absolutely, or by restricting one ingredient, these rats would live longer than their brothers and sisters who were not so restricted. While such work is interesting and valuable in itself, it did not lead on to any definite pointers as to how we might prolong the life-span of the human species.

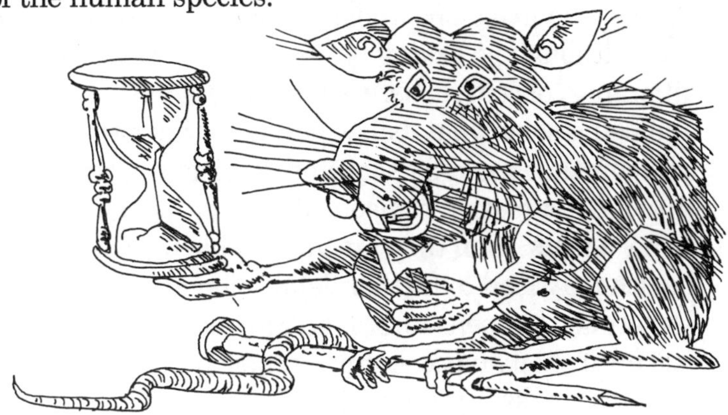

Every species has its own length of life – the group average – and traditionally humans have been supposed to live for 'three-score years and ten'; however, in modern times life expectancy has greatly increased in the developed nations, and we do not know with any surety just what is our 'natural' life-span. In the present state of knowledge, however, as far as diet is concerned, there is absolutely no indication that any special food or food additive will make us live longer. However, there is some evidence that the type of diet that is eaten by Mediterranean people is correlated with a slightly longer life. They consume a great deal of olive oil in place of the fatty meat eaten in the north of Europe, and their diet has a greater vegetable content. The best bet is for you to stick to a good mixed diet, with no fancy additives, and then you will live as long as the programming in your genes intended you to, unless disease or accident leads to an untimely death.

TREAT YOURSELF WITH KINDNESS AND RESPECT

A recent survey showed that about 3% of old people in Britain were malnourished. The causes of such malnourishment were various, but they included poverty, low intelligence, depression, and a lack of proper self-care, and many, if not all, of these factors were inter-related.

People who live alone and are isolated, tend not to eat properly, even although by taking proper care they could do so. There is a difference, of course, between being diagnosed as 'malnourished', and being somewhat below par as to the optimal standard of nourishment that could be achieved. A vicious circle may set in: if through depression someone does not take enough care over his or her meals, then they are vulnerable to illnesses, and such ill-health may lead to further depression and self-neglect. This sometimes happens after men are bereaved if they have never learnt to shop and cook during their married years, and cannot be bothered to do anything other than live off any sort of food that requires no preparation.

The best advice is for you to take care over your meals; make them interesting and varied, and remember that a little of what you fancy does you good – even if it is not always a food approved of by the dieticians. Take an interest in food; ideally you should eat in company, for meals at their best are a social occasion, but when this is not practicable, treat yourself with courtesy and consideration and behave to yourself as you would when offering meals to an honoured guest, even when you are eating alone.

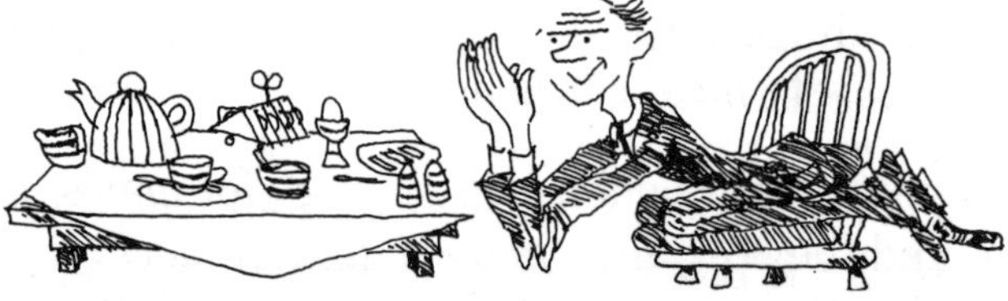

This extra trouble is worth it you will enjoy much better health. While there is every reason to avoid obesity, a condition that carries all sorts of health risks as will be explained in later chapters, you should not aim to be thin, as many younger people do. Thinness in the elderly is not a sign of good health.

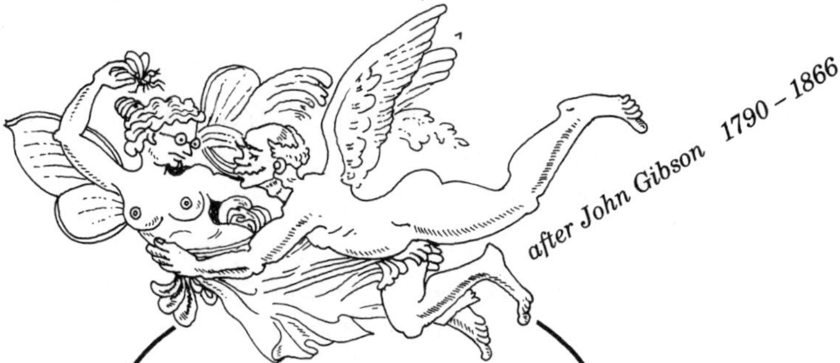

WHAT ABOUT SEX?

Chapter 5

Sexual activity of one sort and another is normal for healthy people, although there is nothing particularly strange about those who just aren't interested. It is usually more important in the younger years of life, and according to the famous *Kinsey Report*, young men are at their peak of 'performance' just before the age of 20, but young women are generally more interested in their 30s. Of course, it depends what is meant by 'performance', and this is a matter that I will discuss later. The sexual drive decreases with age, and the forms it takes change, but expressions of sexuality vary greatly among different people; this is one of the outstanding features of the findings of Kinsey's research which surprised many readers at the time it was published.

The Kinsey studies were published in 1948 (for males) and 1953 (for females) and they certainly made a great impact on public attitudes to sex in the years that followed, although there were many other factors working for the liberalization of social attitudes in the post-war period. The researches of Masters and Johnston in the 1960s also informed the public more about the realities of sexual behaviour, and helped to dispel many ancient misconceptions and prejudices, but at that time very little interest was focused on the sexuality of people over 60 because it was simply assumed that people in later life just weren't interested, and had no sex life at all! It was not until the 1980s that any serious attempt was made to find out about what was normal for older people; one large research study was conducted in the USA with 4,246 men and women aged 50 to 93, by Edward Brecher working for the Consumers' Union. There had been earlier smaller studies by scientists interested in the general health of older people which paved the way to the realization that sexuality does not die out after middle-age and is perfectly natural and normal.

It is extraordinary how the medical profession lent its prestige to bolster up the most absurd misconceptions about sexuality in general, and concerning older people in particular, while they were making considerable headway in the scientific understanding of health and the combating of disease in other ways. One can only suppose that many doctors in the Victorian era, and for the years that followed, were men who were very confused about sexuality themselves. Even the famous Havelock Ellis, who shocked his colleagues at the time by his outspoken writings on sexuality, wrote utter nonsense when he came to write about sexual expression in older people. He dared to contradict older doctors such as William Acton, who denied that young wives had any sexual feelings and taught young men that:

> As a general rule, a modest woman seldom desires any sexual gratification for herself. She submits to her husband, but only to please him; and, but for the desire for maternity, would far rather be relieved of his attentions.

Although Havelock Ellis allowed that young women did have sexual desires, when it came to women after the age of the menopause he appeared to think that any expression of sexual feeling was abnormal and morbid. As for older men he believed that age-related changes in the prostate produced a 'physical irritation' that could lead to a 'flaring up' of sexual desire that impelled them to molest children.

Before describing what really does take place with ageing, it will be best to discuss some of the traditional myths.

MYTHS ABOUT SEXUALITY IN LATER LIFE

1. Intercourse and emission of semen are debilitating and will tend to hasten old age and death.
2. One's sex life can be prolonged by abstinence in earlier years and inactivity in later years.
3. Masturbation is a childish activity that is put aside when one reaches adulthood, and is carried out by older persons only if they are seriously disturbed.
4. Coital satisfaction decreases considerably after the menopause.
5. Older men are particularly subject to sexual deviations, for example, exhibitionism and child molesting.
6. Older women who still enjoy sex were probably nymphomaniacs when they were younger.
7. Most older men lose their ability and desire to have sex.
8. Sexual ability and performance remain the same throughout life.
9. If older individuals go without sex for several years, they will not be able to have sex at a future time.
10. Older people with chronic illness or physical disabilities should cease sex activity completely.

Reprinted by the kind permission of Croft, L H (1982) *Sexuality in Later Life. Appendix B.* Boston: John Wright.

1. The question of debility

All that we know about the physiology of sex makes it quite clear that intercourse and the emission of semen is not debilitating. In later life, men do not manufacture as much semen, just as some other natural secretions are not as copious, and some acts of intercourse are not accompanied by a seminal emission. Nonetheless, they may still have an orgasm, which is an event in the nervous system, and experience the pleasure and relaxation that follows. What evidence we have shows that continued sexual activity is associated with longevity, and it may be that the former promotes the latter, but this is not certain. As in many other things we may be confusing cause with effect. It appears that widowers who re-marry will have longer lives than those who don't, but marriage means a number of things. The re-married widowers may have wives who look after them in various ways, in addition to going to bed with them. It may be that it is the men who are more robust in later life who re-marry, and their general robustness, rather than continued sexual relations, may be the cause of their longevity.

2. The effect of early abstinence

The poet William Blake tells us that:

Abstinence sows sand all over

The ruddy limbs and flaming hair

But desire gratified

Plants fruits of life and beauty there.

As far as there is any evidence, people who begin sexual activity earlier in life continue it later in life. The concept of our having just so much in a store of energy, like petrol in a tank, and when it is used up no more energy is available, is quite mistaken. The saying 'Use it or lose it' is more appropriate here.

3. Masturbation

Some people masturbate all their lives, whether or not they are also engaging in sex with a partner. Masturbation is almost universal among males, particulary when they are young, lusty and lacking sexual partners. Some females claim that they never, or very rarely, masturbate. Many older people who have not got partners masturbate regularly, and it is a healthful way of relieving sexual tension. Some Victorian doctors attributed all sorts of physical and mental ills to masturbation. Lacking any actual evidence for their absurd statements about the consequences of masturbation they often quoted the book of an anonymous clergyman published in 1710, entitled *Onania, or the Heinous Sin of Self-pollution.* It is amazing that even an eminent psychiatrist such as Henry Maudsley, who wrote so wisely on many topics in mental health, should get caught up in the Victorian hysteria against masturbation. The legacy of their spreading of misinformation is with us yet, and some people still believe that masturbation can cause insanity.

Wendy and Sally Greengross in their recent book addressed to older people, *Living, Loving and Ageing* deal with the matter very simply:

> Most people nowadays accept that it is not only harmless, but also enjoyable. It can help people to relax and relieve tension, and release the energy that might otherwise be used in trying to suppress sexual feelings. Everyone has some sexual needs and people who do not have a partner, and often those who do, may nevertheless find pleasure in stimulating themselves sexually.

4. Sex for women after the menopause

For some women the menopause gives rise to a severe deficiency of the hormone oestrogen, and this can cause vaginal dryness and hence pain on intercourse. This can be remedied by hormone replacement therapy, a sophisticated treatment that needs medical monitoring, and in a few cases is not advisable. Vaginal dryness can also be helped by hormone creams or lubricating gel. But for a number of other women no such disability arises, and pleasure in intercourse increases after the menopause, largely for psychological reasons, such as ceasing to have to bother about contraception, and leading a more relaxed style of life because their children are grown up.

In one study of 441 women over 60 the question was asked, 'How does sex feel now compared with when you were younger?' In their answers 41% reported 'better', 40% reported 'the same', and 19% said it was 'worse'. When the same question was asked of 273 men over 60, the replies were 27% 'better', 37% 'the same', and 35% 'worse'. This is rather what we might expect, as in later life women retain their energy rather better than men.

5. Older men molesting children

It is quite untrue that child-molesters tend to be old men, yet the myth was perpetuated even by that relatively enlightened sexologist Havelock Ellis as mentioned earlier. Child-molesters are typically males in their thirties whose sex lives have been warped and stunted possibly by a moralistic upbringing.

6. About these 'nymphomaniacs'

The label 'nymphomaniac' is a silly term of abuse applied to women who enjoy sex and rival men in their ability to go out and get it. Most older women enjoy sex; the sad thing is that many of them are without partners in the later years of life, simply because as we go up the age gradient men die off sooner than women. No-one has yet come up with a satisfactory suggestion as to how this situation can be remedied. It may surprise feminists that the fine old campaigner for women's rights, Betty Friedan, is now advocating polygamy in later life in her most recent book. I think that very few men in later life would contemplate taking on a harem of women, whatever they did in their youth!

7. Older men having no interest in sex

It is not true that men have no interest in sex when they are old. Various surveys involving thousands of men have shown that in the great majority of older men interest in sex is maintained. Their 'ability' in terms of penile potency, declines with age, just as their ability to run round the block and other physical achievements decline, but lovemaking is not simply a matter of copulation.

8. About sexual ability

The myth as stated is very strange, and is the converse of the one mentioned before. As far as men are concerned I think the myth can only be believed by women who have had very little experience of the male sex, for every man knows how most of his physical abilities wane with age. Men function differently when they are older, and some men say that their sex lives are better in later life, but being 'better' does not mean that they are more potent as lovers, but that they get more satisfaction out of their sex lives.

As far as women are concerned, there may be some truth in the statement, for some women have fallen in love very late in life, and having found a satisfactory sexual partner they report that their response and fulfilment is greater than when they were young.

9. The alleged inability to resume a sex life

In general this is not true either for men or for women, but if individuals have become discouraged and believe themselves to be 'past it', they may have difficulty in resuming a sex life for psychological reasons even when the opportunity occurs. A lot depends upon people's self-image, but finding the right partner at any age does wonders for the self-image.

10. Ceasing sexual activity because of illness and disability

The fear of doing oneself an injury by copulating is common. On the contrary, the maintenance of sexual activity keeps up the morale of a sick or injured person and responsible authorities have been concerned with advising handicapped and sick people how best they may adapt to their disabilities and continue to make love.

Fear of self-harm by copulation is very common among those who have had heart attacks, and again I quote from Wendy and Sally Greengross:

> As people live longer they are more likely to suffer from some deterioration to their cardiac efficiency and some people get 'heart attacks'. Twenty or thirty years ago they would have expected to spend the rest of their lives as a cardiac invalid. Nowadays, however, people are encouraged to return to full activity as soon as possible. Generally it is accepted that anyone who can walk up two flights of stairs can easily manage sexual intercourse, and as sex is an enjoyable activity, it should be resumed as soon as the couple wish.*

A GENERAL OVERVIEW

Having disposed of the common myths about sex and ageing, let us now consider what really does happen to the sexuality of men and women as they age. First, it should be noted that there are enormous differences between individuals in this matter. Kinsey noted that it was impossible to say what sexual practices, frequencies, etc were 'normal' as people varied so greatly. This is especially true with regard to age, some fifty-year-olds apparently running out of steam while other people in their nineties are still making love. It will be convenient to consider the effect of the ageing process for the two sexes separately.

---

* I have dealt with the problems of sexuality in later life in considerable detail in my book *The Emotional and Sexual Lives of Older People,* published by Chapman & Hall, 1992, to which interested readers are referred.

MEN

Some men tend to suffer from an over-emphasis on physical prowess all their lives; as they age they become less athletic, and this, of course, is manifest in their sexual behaviour as well as everything else. Such men may begin to worry secretly about sexual ageing even as early as their 30s, when they compare their present level of sexual activity with their previous performance as teenagers and in their early 20s. One change that takes place is that the male orgasm does not take place so quickly, but for many couples this is a positive advantage, since the act of copulation may be prolonged by the older man, giving his partner repeated orgasms if this is desired.

As people vary so enormously in their love-making style, no-one can compare themselves with a given norm; all one can do is to compare present with past performance. If you realize the general truth – that love-making in one form or another may continue for the whole of your life, if you feel like it, then you will be reassured and will not become prey to neurotic anxiety.

A man in his teens may have liked to have intercourse several times a night, but by the age of 40 the frequency may be very much reduced – but does it matter? Is he really getting less satisfaction out of his sex life? It may be that the three times a night performance was really to show his partner what a virile lover he was, but now 25 years later, he is more secure in his masculine role and doesn't need to show off, and he may now give himself and his partner more satisfaction than in his teen-age years. When he is in his seventies, a week or more may sometimes pass without a single act of intercourse, but he may still make love in other ways, such love-making being a steady part of an ongoing erotic relationship. His masculine self-image suffers no diminution because he makes love like a seventy-year-old and not like a teenager.

A ribald joke relates how a sex researcher was conducting a lecture, and having ascertained that every single member of the audience was currently having a sex life, began to ask about frequencies; 'Seven nights a week?' Three hands went up. 'Four or more times a week?' Twelve hands went up. 'Once or twice a week?' Twenty hands went up. And so it went on, just one individual indicating that he had intercourse only once a month. The lecturer noticed that in the front there was a grinning individual who had never put up his hand at all. 'You sir, you seem very pleased with yourself, but I didn't see you raise your hand at all. Tell me, please, how frequently do you have intercourse?' 'Once a year,' the happy man replied, 'But it's tonight!'

If men are ignorant about what will happen to them as they get older they may make both themselves and their partners miserable about sex, give the whole thing up, and be reconciled to being sexless oldies, retired from the battle of life. There is no reason at all why you should have a sex life, as long as you and your partner are happy about it. What a 'sex life' is must be interpreted very broadly, and plenty of partners are perfectly happy and content with just cuddling and other forms of affectionate physical contact. The great majority of men in their 70s cannot expect to continue to lead the same sort of sex life that they did in their 40s. They should realize the nature of the normal age-related changes that take place in both men and women. In general, people don't expect to continue to make love in the same way as they did in middle-age, but they are often very unsure as to what will happen as they continue to get older.

Male 'impotence'

Some men fear that they will become 'impotent' after the age of about 50 or 60, and here they may be a prey to some scare advertising that has been appearing in the press in recent years. A commercial firm that advertises its services for preserving or restoring 'potency' makes the following misleading statement in its publicity brochure:

> Thanks to a revolutionary breakthrough male impotence can now be successfully treated in nine cases out of ten.
>
> This distressing condition is more common than most people imagine. Ten per cent of all men are affected and up to 40% of those over the age of 50.

This is scare advertising, intended to frighten people into coming for treatment and paying out big fees. To claim that 'ten per cent of all men are affected' is virtually meaningless. First, they don't define 'impotence'; is it failure to achieve or maintain erection on all occasions, or one occasion in ten, or one in 100? Second, to say that 'up to 40% of those over the age of 50', are affected, is rubbish. What does 'up to' mean? The percentage affected depends upon the particular age group that is being studied. Finally, it is absurd to make a claim that successful treatment can be given to 'nine cases out of ten'. This certainly would not be true if all their clients were in their 90s! The treatment this clinic offers, according to their publicity brochure, is 'Pharmacologically Induced Penile Erection' which probably means the injection of papavervine or similar agents into the penis, a technique that may have considerable dangers, and may need continued and expensive medical monitoring.

Men who don't properly understand what's happening to them in the normal course of ageing, may fear that they are becoming 'impotent' simply because they experience one or two incidents of failure to achieve erection on a sexual encounter. Such a fear may very well produce performance anxiety which can cause psychogenic impotence. But occasional incidents of unexplained failure to achieve erection happen to some people at all ages, and do not mean very much.

Ovid the great Latin poet wrote an amusing poem on the subject of an episode of 'impotence' he experienced:

Perhaps she did not kiss me as she should,
Nor used the sleight and cunning which she could.
No! She could oaks and adamant have stirred,
And her sweet words deaf boulders would have heard.
Worthy she was to stir all living men,
But neither was I man nor living then . . .
But notwithstanding, like one dead it lay,
Drooping more than a rose plucked yesterday.
Now, when he should not be, he's bolt upright
And craves his task and seeks to have his fight.
Lie down in shame and see you stir no more!
You've caught me with your promises before.
You've tricked me, got me captured weaponless,
And I've endured great shame and sore distress.
Nay, the wench did not disdain a whit
To take it in her hand and play with it.
But when she saw it would by no means stand
But still drooped down, regarding not her hand,
'Why mock me so', she cried, 'or if you're ill,
Who bade you lie down here against your will?
Either you've been bewitched and you're half dead,
Or you came jaded from some other's bed.'

Poor Ovid could not account for his sudden failure of potency, and attributed it to witchcraft. All men may be subject to such occasional failures of potency, especially in later life, and science has not come up with any better explanation than witchcraft!

WOMEN

Not only do men need to know what physiological changes they may expect to take place in their own bodies, and how to cope with them, but they need to understand what happens to women in order to be effective and considerate lovers. Most men probably underestimate the capacity for enjoyment and sexual performance in older women. They are aware that their own sexual performance is declining, and so expect a comparable decline to take place in women, which is not the case. They may not know that if a decline in sexual capacity in women follows the menopause, this may be due to a lack of the hormone oestrogen, a condition that can generally be rectified quite easily by hormone replacement therapy. It's worth repeating that some women enjoy sex more after the menopause.

Women also need to know about men. In their younger years they may have come to regard men as robust and ever-ready studs, who could be expected to do all the wooing to arouse the conventionally reluctant female. In later life the roles may become somewhat reversed in this respect, the sexuality of the woman being the more robust, and that of the man more subject to subtle psychological influences. Sometimes the sex instruction manuals that are written for younger adults make statements that aren't quite true for older people. One such manual states:

> A woman's desire and responsiveness tends to be even more susceptible to psychological influences, internal and external, than a man's. As the saying goes,'Biology moves her but psychology rules her'.

Allowing for the fact that there are enormous individual differences, this male/female contrast is less true in later life, and in many cases the reverse is true, older women being tougher. They live, on average, seven years longer than men, are less upset by bereavement of a spouse, and their sexual capacity doesn't decline with age to the same extent as men's. Their trouble is that there just aren't enough men in their age group, and many of the men who are around are just too timorous and emotionally uncertain of themselves to get involved in a sexual relationship.

Some men give up making love because they feel that they cannot live up to their previous standards of performance, and this creates a most unfortunate social situation. If older men fear the 'challenge' of a situation in which their sexual potency will be put to the test, then they may withdraw from socialization with women, as well as from sexual encounters with them, and this exacerbates a problem that already exists – that there are already four times as many single women as single men after the age of 65. Unless both men and women in the later years of life have adequate knowledge about sexuality, the relations between the two sexes are beset with pitfalls – pitfalls that have been created by the Victorian anti-sex tradition, and the power struggle that seeks to relegate 'the old' to an inferior position in society. This is not a sex-instruction manual; readers who want to gain more detailed knowledge of the subject are referred to the books listed in Appendix B.

WHAT SEXUALITY MEANS IN LATER LIFE

What do we mean by sexuality anyway? This is by no means as simple a question as it seems. Writers like Freud caused a furore in their day by attributing sexuality to the motivation and behaviour of infants, and interpreting much adult behaviour in terms of 'sex'. As there are many problems associated with the continuance of sexual activity in later life, or its renewal after a period of celibacy following bereavement, it may be asked why should not older people just resign themselves to living celibate lives in some circumstances? If they are married, or living in a long-term relationship, they could carry on for the sake of companionship, but not worry if the physical aspect of the relationship comes to a complete end. If they find themselves rendered single, should they aspire to form new sexual relationships ? After all, it's admitted that the physiological drive for sex dies down in intensity with age, at least with men, and it may seem that there is little point in 'stoking', as it were, rather than damping down, a 'furnace' that can lead to all sorts of social inconveniences.

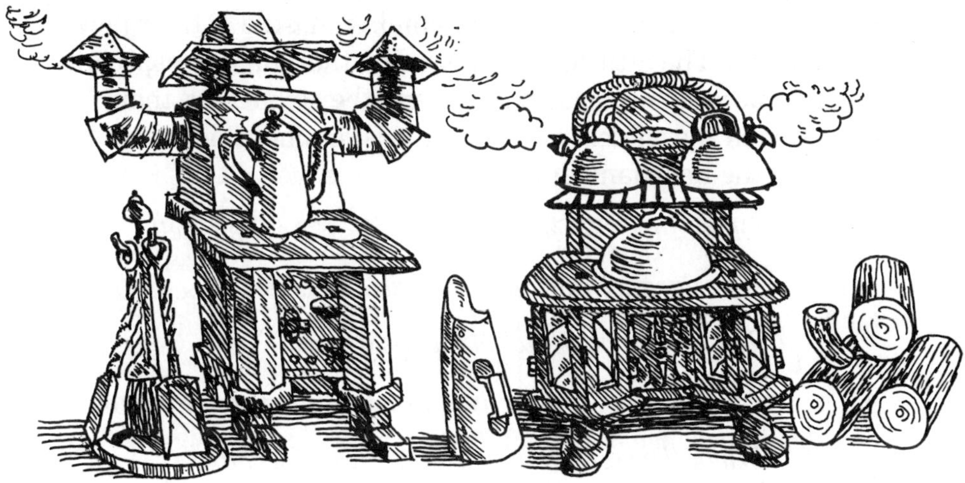

It's entirely understandable if some people see the situation in these terms, especially if they have a vested interest in discouraging the older generation from having any sex lives. Many of those in administrative positions, such as the matrons of old people's homes, would find it more convenient if all their charges were docile, sex-less beings. Similarly, some doctors and social workers might be happier if their older patients and clients would be reconciled to living celibate lives and hence not worry them with problems related to sexuality.

Middle-aged children may sometimes resent signs of continued sexuality in their parents who are rendered single in later life, as this may lead to re-marrying and hence a possible division of the inheritance. There is also the question of sheer emotional jealousy that may be shown by middle-aged children if a widowed parent contemplates acquiring a new partner. This is especially true if the child is unhappily married, or has failed to find a suitable partner, and such jealousy can be extreme.

I was once the guest on a TV show devoted to older parents rendered single in later life who were contemplating marrying a new partner, and they came with their children hostile to their new relationship. The attitudes expressed by the children, especially the men, were sometimes extreme, and they expressed their opposition in the wildest of terms. I was reminded of Hamlet's speech in the Bedchamber scene:

Oh shame! Where is thy blush? Rebellious hell,

If thou canst mutine in a matron's bones

To flaming youth let virtue be as wax,

And melt in her own fire: proclaim no shame

When the compulsive ardour gives the charge,

Since frost itself as actively does burn,

And reason panders will.

Yet in this play Hamlet's mother was evidently about 40. His resentment of his mother's re-marriage had many sources, yet here it took the form of sexual jealousy – *Go not to my uncle's bed!*

Is it right, the jealous ones may say, for organizations such as Age Concern to encourage the grandparent generation to expect to lead a full sex life? Will the old things never give up?

To answer this question, it is necessary to explain a concept of sexuality that applies in later life, and is rather different from that which characterizes the younger years of adulthood. Most older people may take some time fully to realize the physiological and psycho-social changes that will take place over perhaps the last 30 years of their lives, and if they hope to recapture precisely the same sort of sexual satisfactions that they had in youth and middle-age, they will be disappointed. Yet sexuality in later life can be fulfilling and of great importance to many people, although some at all ages seem to lead well-adjusted asexual lives. It takes all sorts to make a world!

To retain a healthy self-concept, people need to regard themselves positively with regard to their feminine or masculine sexuality. This is generally a deep psychological need, and denial of it may lead to depression and preternatural ageing. As people age, they are subject to subtle psycho-social changes, as well as physiological changes. If a man tries to cling to a macho image of being a frequent and efficient phallic performer in his later decades of life, he might as well try to compete in the athletic contests he used to go in for half a century before. With unrealistic expectations he'll be heading for trouble, and may perhaps suffer from performance anxiety, so that eventually he comes to regard himself as 'impotent', and withdraws from love-making altogether. But with a more sophisticated understanding of the expression of emotional feeling in physical terms, he may enjoy a lifetime of rewarding love-making in which phallic performance, appropriate to his age, need not play a major part. With a woman, the problem is different, but there's no reason why she should ever lose her sense of femininity, or to cease to be attractive to the right person despite her growing wrinkles.

For many people, 'sex' means copulation with the goal of the male orgasm, conceived as the ejaculation of semen. Although most intercourse is engaged in not for procreation but for recreation, this goal tends to be greatly over-emphasised. However, this traditional view of sex is becoming modified in more recent years, partly due to the feminist movement, but also due to the work of sex-researchers and therapists. When sex-therapists have asked people what they really want of sex, the answer appears to be pleasure, satisfaction, psychological contentment, a sense of self-worth and a celebration of their love for their partner. It has been pointed out that the language which many people use in referring to sexual activity emphasises the 'getting to' rather than the 'experiencing of' a pleasurable activity. The terms 'foreplay' and 'afterplay' emphasise that there's a 'big event', a goal which has to be reached, and all else is subsidiary. Some feminists have complained angrily of the male definition of sex – that it lasts 'until he comes' – and then it is all over! The emphasis on penovaginal intercourse culminating in male orgasm as being the essential and defining characteristic of love-making, is regarded by many as merely fulfilling a macho male need to boost their egos. Investigations of female sexuality have shown that many women's feelings of fulfilment in sex depended on a far broader range of activities involving intimate sexual techniques. Some women have never experienced orgasm in intercourse, but experience it regularly or occasionally through other contacts in love-making.

One of the greatest insights that an ageing man can achieve is to realize that his masculinity doesn't depend wholly on his phallic prowess, and that an experienced lover will be able to give and receive sensual pleasure and emotional satisfaction through the wide range of love-making techniques that are generally known by sex- therapists as 'pleasuring'. The misconception that 'foreplay' is something that the man does to the woman just in order to get her ready for him to penetrate her needs correction. Rather, the more satisfactory aim is to achieve a level of physical and emotional interaction between the couple. Whether or not this involves peno-vaginal intercourse later on, is another matter. Some quite young couples go in for what they call 'non-penetrative sex'. There are no musts in love-making. Some couples achieve their sexual pleasure without actual copulation.

Older men should ask themselves 'What do I need sex for – is it a compulsive effort to demonstrate to myself and others that I am not yet a worn out 'old man' ?' Many people use the rituals of love-making for purposes that are basically asexual, and this is pretty pointless. Some researchers have found that even among younger people, many women enjoy the total experience involving all sorts of caressing. We may call this 'fore-play', but it doesn't necessarily come before anything.

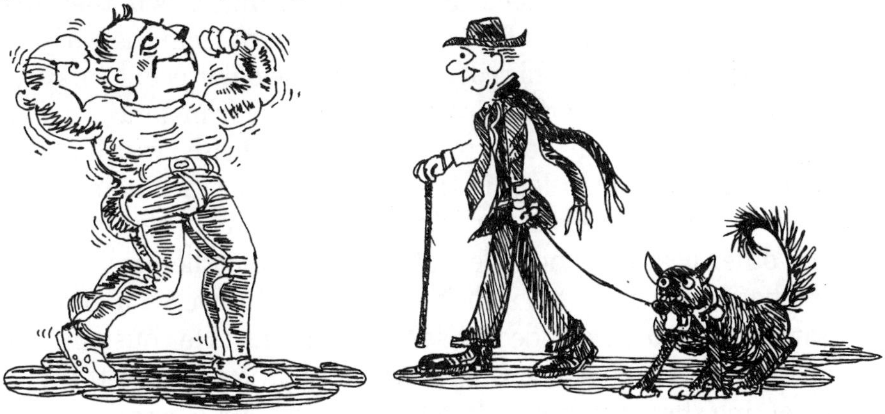

Younger men tend to say that the act of intercourse is more important to them, but this may reflect a strong psychological as well as a physical need, and it may not apply to older lovers if they are happy about their male identity and feel no need to prove themselves.

Women sometimes get a raw deal if their male partner, finding that his phallic performance is declining with age, withdraws entirely from all sexual encounters out of pride. She may be still as ready for love-making in all its aspects as she ever was, but she may have to endure a total deprivation for many years because of her husband's 'impotence'. This cruel deprivation may be interpreted by her as being all her fault, attributing it to her ageing appearance, and some men will give this as a reason for their withdrawal from sexual relations.

DO OLDER PEOPLE NEED ADDITIONAL INFORMATION?

Many men and women in later life may be perfectly content with whatever form their sexual expression has taken over a number of years, or they may be healthy and happy with no sex life at all, but others may welcome additional information which relieves them of guilt and pressure to perform to an unrealistic standard. It's liberating to realize that there are enormous natural variations between individuals, and between couples, as to their expression of sexuality, as first became apparent from the early studies of Kinsey and his colleagues. Some older people may need liberating from all sorts of irrational taboos: for instance, a woman in her seventies may begin to suffer from arthritis, which makes it painful to spread her legs in the face-to-face position of intercourse that she has enjoyed all her adult life. She may never have used any other position, and indeed, have regarded other positions (if she has heard of them!) as being somewhat 'perverse' and not within the province of decent sexual relations. Her husband may be too shy to urge her to vary their usual practice, regretfully accepting that they must abandon all intercourse because of her arthritis. It needs to be pointed out to such a couple that their difficulty may be solved by using other techniques and positions, and that they are neither 'perverse' nor uncommon. Similarly, all sorts of sexual techniques that are described in modern sex-instruction books that younger people practise for fun and for variety, are very suitable for older people whose minor disabilities make the continuance of their usual forms of love-making more difficult.

Here we come to one of the great difficulties in imparting knowledge to many, although not to all, older people. Some may say, in effect, 'But surely such antics are only for the young – it would be unseemly for us to behave in such a way, or even to discuss it together!'

THE SHYNESS OF MANY OLDER PEOPLE

The following incident illustrates a very real problem. At a recent international conference convened by a group of the University of the Third Age, there were various eminent speakers lecturing on topics of special interest to older people. It was announced that many of these speakers had books of their authorship on display and available at a nearby bookshop, and attenders at the conference were invited to go there, browse, and buy them. These books attracted some attention, and there was quite a sale of them, with the exception of one author. This was Alex Comfort, whose talk at the conference was much appreciated, but only two books of his authorship were displayed in the bookshop, *The Joy of Sex* and *More Joy of Sex*, and these were left severely alone. These two books contain some sensible facts and advice on ageing, but they are lavishly and quite tastefully illustrated with drawings of young and comely men and women making love in a great variety of ways, and this was enough to put off older people from buying them openly, or to be seen reading them in a bookshop.

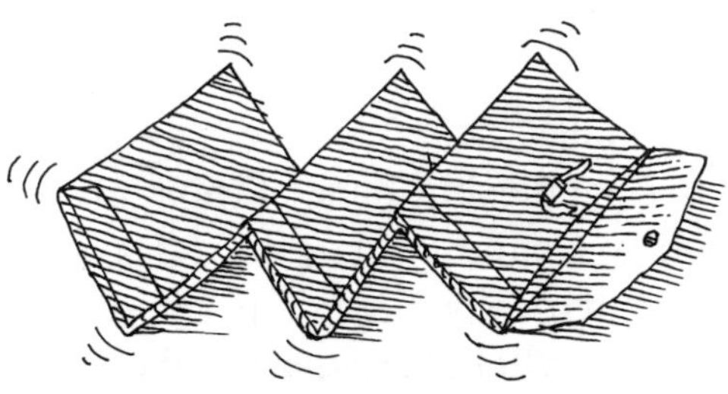

I know a woman in her 60s who has one of them in a brown envelope in her desk, whereas a younger woman might display it openly on her bookshelf, without giving much thought to its presence. The older generation still have a struggle with the taboos of the Victorian past.

In a book published by Age Concern, *Living, Loving and Ageing*, there is a humorous cartoon showing the notice board of an old people's home asking people to sign up for various activities – knitting, recipe swop, bingo, pottery, and kamasutra. While each activity attracts a few ticks, it is the kamasutra class that attracts a whole cluster of ticks, and an old lady is shown adding hers. This may represent the wish, rather than the reality, but it would be interesting to see how such an offer was received if it were really included among the other voluntary classes and activities in such a home.

It is difficult, therefore, to get the older generation to buy, borrow or read books of sex instruction. They are embarrassed to be reading such books at their age, and whether or not they are interested in them, they pretend that they don't need them. In the 1920s and 1930s when such books came widely on the market, they were often sold in 'rubber goods' shops, along with condoms, douches and Damerroids, or sold in back-street bookshops which dealt in surreptitious pornography, and they may still retain this image in the minds of many older people. The fact that Dr Comfort's sex books are now attractively presented and sold openly in respectable bookshops is all to the good, but their bold appeal to the young makes older people shy of reading them.

Comfort's re-issued paperback *A Good Age* is well illustrated with pictures of older people, but none of them are making love. It has a good section on sexuality in ageing. The Age Concern book mentioned above which is directed to the reading public is mainly about the sex lives of older people and offers much sensible advice.

Several useful books on this topic are listed in Appendix B. The giving of advice about sexual health to older people often falls to doctors and other health-care workers, and Karen Hawton makes the point that:

It is unwise to assume that a couple have a sophisticated knowledge of sexuality; very often a couple who give this impression will be unwilling to admit to areas of ignorance, or be unaware of their blindspots. A fairly didactic educational session, in which pictures are used, is helpful. This session should be tailored to needs and problems, as well as the educational level, of the individual couple.

The paradox here is that more educated and superficially sophisticated people may be the ones more prone to pretend to a greater knowledge of sexuality than they possess, whereas less educated men and women may freely admit to the extent of their ignorance.

The following case may be of help and encouragement to others. A widowed lady in her 60s came to live in a new town and went to register with a local doctor, who naturally asked her about all matters relating to her health. As this lady had an artificial hip the doctor offered to give her advice as to how she might manage sexual intercourse in a comfortable position. The lady expressed surprise at this, and reiterated that she was a widow and never expected to have intercourse again 'at her age'. Some time later this widow fell in love with a man and formed a very satisfactory sexual partnership with him, so with some embarrassment she went back to the doctor and asked for the advice she had previously not wished to hear!

As far as your health is concerned, therefore, remember that it is never too late to fall in love, and that in sexual matters, as with much else in life, a little of what you fancy does you good.

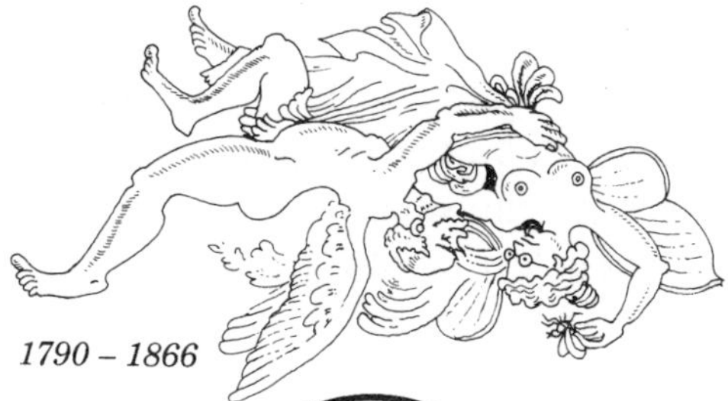

after after John Gibson 1790 – 1866

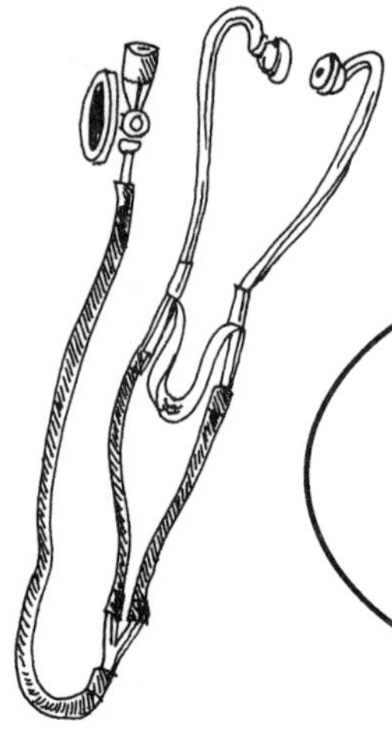

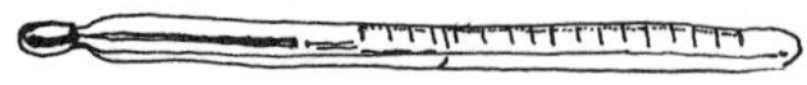

Chapter 6

YOU AND YOUR DOCTOR

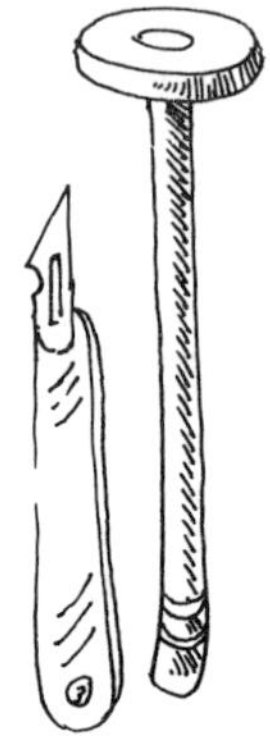

HOLD THE PHYSICIAN IN HONOUR FOR HE IS ESSENTIAL TO YOU,
AND GOD IT WAS WHO ESTABLISHED HIS PROFESSION.
FROM GOD THE DOCTOR HAS HIS WISDOM.
THUS GOD'S CREATIVE WORK CONTINUES WITHOUT CEASE.
HE WHO IS A SINNER TOWARD HIS MAKER WILL BE DEFIANT TOWARD HIS DOCTOR.

The above notice is posted on the wall of a physician's surgery in a small town in Ohio, but I don't suppose that many doctors demand such compliance from their patients elsewhere. It is true that on the dustcover of an American book on the health-care of older people there is a photograph of a little old lady in a posture of adoration and gratitude caressing her doctor's hand. One commentator on this book says, 'Practitioners familiar with the health care of the elderly recognize that this is as much an erroneous stereotype as another possible picture of a little old lady angrily whacking a doctor over the head with cane'. However, both stereotypes exist and the cartoon shown below presents a view of doctors held by some elderly women.

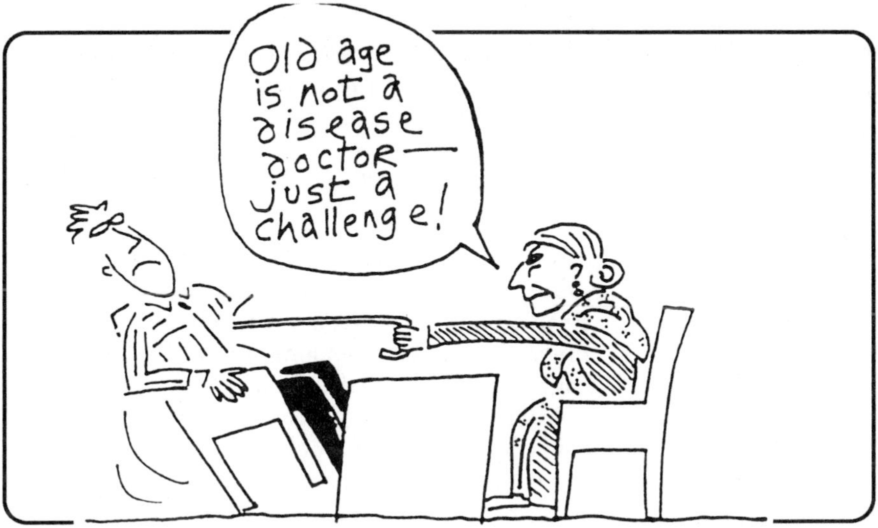

Cartoon reproduced with permission from the artist, Angela Martin, and the publishers, Piatkus Books, from *Growing Old Disgracefully.*

DIFFERENT TYPES OF PATIENT

It has been suggested that there are two types of patients, the 'physician-dependent' and the 'fiercely independent'. Obviously what has been depicted above represents caricatures of two extreme types: the lady who expresses doggy devotion and gratitude and the one who challenges her doctor's authority with extreme vigour. Nevertheless, it will be helpful to discuss these two types.

The physician-dependent patient

The physician-dependent patient eschews self-care, and acts as though his or her health is entirely the responsibility of the doctor. In medical writings there are often debates about how to deal with 'noncompliant' patients, that is, patients who quietly deceive their GPs by not taking the medicines prescribed for them, and secretly flout the recommendations for their conduct, such as continuing to drink spirits when the treatment involves abstinence. Physician-dependent people are certainly not lacking in compliance, in fact they may be over-compliant, but they are by no means ideal patients from the doctor's point of view. In dealing with such cases Dr Andrew Malleson has this to say:

> The doctor-patient relationship, as with any other helper-helpee interaction often turns out to be the most unhelpful of all kinds of human relationships. Problems are problems, but they also have their uses. Once it becomes the doctor's responsibility to solve the patient's problems, the patient can comfortably keep them. It is not his fault if they do not get solved, it is the doctor's. In my experience as a doctor, often the easiest way to make a patient angry is to deny my competence to help. It is of course not my modesty that makes him angry, but the fact that by doing so, I pass the responsibility of doing something about his problems back to him. If he does not solve them it is not my fault but his, and he can no longer continue to live with his problems comfortably.

The above practitioner's complaint refers, of course, to the psychological aspects of medical treatment. All disorders have both a physical and a psychological component and the physician-dependent patient comes more and more to expect the doctor to be a counsellor, father confessor and big brother. Sometimes the medical problems seem to be almost an excuse for coming for comfort and support. In later life it is not uncommon to have all sorts of minor disabilities; if we are active and busy they are hardly noticed, but in conditions of underactivity, loneliness and depression such disabilities may become painful and even crippling.

Because of the large number of elderly people in the community nowadays, about 15% of the older population are utilizing 25% of the medical care; it is arguable that if so many people in later life were not compulsorily thrown out of work ('retired'), rendered impoverished, and relatively socially isolated by the very nature of our society, such a large percentage of medical care would not need to be given to them.

One of the effects of the behaviour of physician-dependent patients is that the doctor, repeatedly asked to show loving care and to cure situations that arise simply from battered self-esteem, loneliness, under-activity, and boredom, feels that the only possible reaction is to reach for the prescription pad and hand out a totally unnecessary drug.

The 'fiercely independent' patient

Patients of this type do not like going to the doctor, as it implies that they are not competent to handle their own affairs. They tend to mistrust doctors, and if they are practically forced to see their GP through some emergency they are not always willing to be quite frank about their ailments and their life-style. The doctor, aware that the patient is not perhaps telling the whole story, must depend on the results of physiological laboratory tests and signs that emerge from physical examination.

Such patients may be very mistrustful of any drugs prescribed. They know all about placebos, and may suspect that they are being fobbed of with some inert substance just to stop them moaning, or to cover up the doctor's incompetence to make a proper diagnosis of their complaint. They may be equally suspicious of active drugs, and argue that it is wrong and unnatural to swallow any 'foreign' substance that may do the body untold harm. Such patients may have a fund of stories about medical incompetence. Elderly patients may have very long memories and treasure horror stories to back up their general distrust of doctors. In one study of patients in a residential area it was the older people who complained most: a third of those over the age of 60 reported at least one episode of medical error, ranging from doctors giving insufficient information to mistakes that actually caused harm to patients, even though these incidents occurred many years ago. For instance, one elderly respondent recalled that 28 years ago a doctor had diagnosed her husband's stomach cancer as sinus trouble, and he died of it. Another reported, 'Twenty years ago my brother felt run down and our doctor told him it was his teeth so he had them all out – but he still felt run down, so he went to another doctor and they found he had TB.' Even trivial incidents of mis-diagnosis that happened nearly half a century ago were remembered and advanced as evidence that doctors cannot be trusted!

Medical practice has changed considerably over more recent decades, and younger doctors must feel that they are operating under an unfair cloud of suspicion created by the less competent of their profession many years ago, and enshrouded in the long memories of their older patients.

While the 'fiercely independent' patients tend to be highly suspicious of all drugs because they are chosen by the doctors and not themselves, they can be real suckers for the huge range of herbal and 'natural' medicines that are now so widely available in 'health' shops, even though these are remarkably expensive. They feel that if they shop around and use their own discretion their ailments are under their own control, even though they may never succeed in finding a remedy that works.

I knew an elderly lady who developed severe eczema and at last consented to go and see her doctor about it. The doctor prescribed one of the many drugs that are used in the treatment of this condition, and on the first day of taking this medicine she felt unpleasantly drowsy, but instead of going back to the doctor and asking for the treatment to be varied, having had her anti-medical suspicions confirmed, she went to a herbalist shop and bought an ointment based on marigold flowers. When the marigold ointment was used up, with no improvement in her eczema, she switched to another herbal ointment, and then to another, but I do not think she ever got rid of her eczema.

While the 'physician-dependent' type of patient is one sort of pest to doctors, the 'fiercely independent' type is another. The doctor is never sure that the whole story of the ailment has been told, particularly if it relates to some foolish or undignified behaviour on the part of the sufferer. There also remains some uncertainty as to whether medicines are really being taken or recommended regimes are being followed. A consultant geriatrician wrote to me recently saying:

> I think it would be useful to stress . . . the need for negotiations between lay and medical persons with regard to lifestyle issues which may or may not be acceptable to modification by the individual. By this I mean whether or not they are prepared to give up smoking, whether or not they are prepared to reduce alcohol intake, and whether or not they find taking pills unacceptable. Honesty from doctor to patient is, I think, taken as a part of good medical practice, but equally honesty from patients to the medical profession is also important – perhaps this is best paraphrased as, 'I hear what you are saying doctor, but I do not like the message and therefore I will choose to ignore it, but you ought to know that I am doing that, rather than me trying to pull the wool over your eyes, and pretend that I am taking your advice.'

Perhaps the most unfortunate aspect of over-independence on the part of patients is that as they are reluctant to visit any doctor, particularly when they suspect that some aspect of their life-style may be criticised. They go on postponing seeking advice while a serious condition may be steadily developing, hoping that by their own efforts it will be overcome, perhaps by the application of 'home remedies' or over-the-counter medicines that seem appropriate.

When eventually the condition has become so serious that friends or family insist that medical advice is sought, the doctor is faced with an ailment that could have been checked or cured in its early stages, but is now so serious that the chances of effective treatment are slim. I have known personally two cases of death from cancers that might have been checked if they had had proper attention in their early stages, but the sufferers were of such an independent temperament that they refused to admit that they needed medical treatment until it was too late.

The happy medium

Two contrasted types of people have been described and I am not suggesting that they are so very common in their extreme form. Throughout this book I am insisting that your health is your own responsibility and not your doctor's, but while enumerating the evils of over-dependence that make a reasonable patient-doctor relationship impossible, it is as well to have considered how the relationship may be damaged by the extreme of the opposite approach.

It must be admitted that the great improvement in the nation's health and the extension of life expectancy has been achieved principally by public health measures involving better sanitation, housing, diet, and all kinds of preventive medicine such as widespread vaccination, rather than the clinical medicine of the doctors' surgeries.

Nevertheless, in order to maintain a healthy life in your later years a good working relationship with your GP is essential. The less often you need to see your doctor the better, although after the age of 75 an annual check-up is advisable, even though you may feel perfectly well, and after examining you and consulting your medical records your doctor will be in a better position to put things right if anything threatens to become a problem.

If your doctor is to be of maximum use to you he must know something about you, your life style and your attitude to illness. The great British physician and teacher, Sir William Osler, said, 'It is more important to know what sort of patient has a disease than what sort of disease a patient has.' While this is a gross exaggeration which no-one takes literally, it expresses an important principle – that a good GP gets to know some salient facts about his patients. As one medical writer has expressed it, 'There is little point in a doctor X-raying his patient's neck when it is his mother-in-law and not his cervical spine that gives him the pain.' This approach leads to what is known as 'holistic medicine', in which the doctor attempts to treat the 'whole person' rather than just the disorder of which the patient complains. As with most movements, some medical devotees may go rather far in their interpretation of how patients should be treated holistically. The hang-over from Dr Freud's teaching may lead a doctor to try to interpret a patient's simple disorder as symbolic of some underlying psychic complex – should a doctor really refrain from x-raying a man's neck because he suspects that his mother-in-law is a 'pain in the neck'? Anyway, as the doctor cannot cure the patient of his domestic incubus, he might as well get busy with the neck which he may possibly do something for.

Many patients may reasonably object to their GP trying to 'psych' them: a woman who goes to the surgery with a sprained ankle may feel it quite inappropriate to be questioned about her sex life by an over enthusiastic holistic practitioner. What do you do about it if you find yourself in this predicament? The answer is simple – point out to the doctor your objections and if they are not treated sympathetically, change to another doctor as you have a perfect right to.

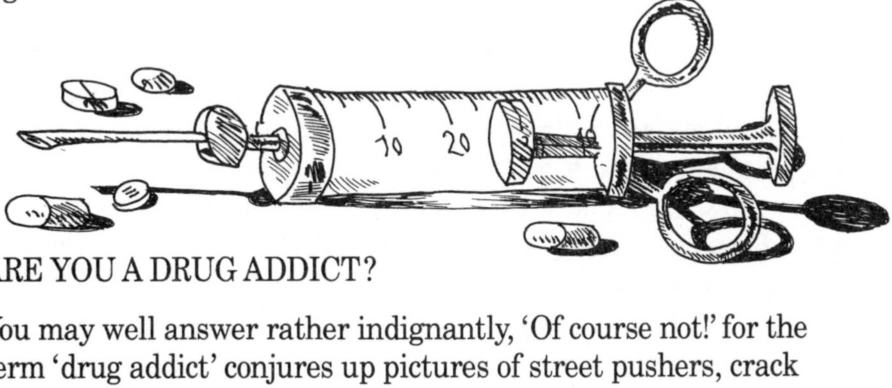

ARE YOU A DRUG ADDICT?

You may well answer rather indignantly, 'Of course not!' for the term 'drug addict' conjures up pictures of street pushers, crack merchants, and addicts with dirty syringes. But the plain fact is that an alarming number of older people are consuming enormous quantities of drugs and are addicted to a habit which is nonetheless dangerous because the drugs are legally prescribed. The medical profession as a whole deplore this but they feel rather helpless in the situation that has grown up.

The history of drug usage in the NHS is very interesting, especially as it affects older people. When the National Health Service was introduced in Britain in 1948 all drugs on prescription became free, but there had already been established a pattern of doctors coping with their patients' demands by reaching for the prescription pad. At that date most of the drugs were not very effective and therefore not very harmful in their side effects. What has increased by leaps and bounds is the expense of drugs. In the 1960s 100 aspirins could be bought at the chemists for about 5 pence; the cost today is about £1.00. In addition to such a simple drug as aspirin there are many designer drugs produced today that are very expensive indeed, and what is spent on the enormous national drug bill detracts from what could be devoted to other services in the NHS.

In 1956 the Conservative government introduced prescription charges to try to check the ever-growing public appetite for drugs; the later Labour government abolished this charge, true to the original conception of free medical care, but were forced to introduce it at an even higher rate in 1968.

Since then there have been successive increases which have at least served to check the ever-growing volume of medicines being swallowed by the working population – but not by the pensioners who, receiving the drugs free, have steadily demanded more and more. Now about one-third of the prescribed drugs are consumed by retired people. If it really kept them fit and free from recurrent illnesses there would be some sense in this expenditure, but for some time there have been published disturbing reports about drug-induced disorders among elderly people.

One such report describes a survey of geriatric units in which adverse reactions to prescribed drugs were a contributory cause leading to hospital admission in 12.4% of the cases.

One of the major problems is that the impressive armamentarium of drugs now available to the medical profession has been developed and established with reference to the adult population, with special caveats about using them for children under a certain age. So far little research has been done concerning their effect on people over a certain age. Normal ageing is accompanied by changes and deterioration in many physiological functions.

Older people differ from younger both in their reactions to drugs and the way in which their bodies eliminate them from the system. Many common drugs that are given to elderly people, such as digoxin for heart trouble and antibiotics to fight acute infections, are not excreted by the kidneys at the same rate as is normal for younger people, and there is therefore the possibility of them building up into a dangerously high level in the system. Another factor that is a cause for concern is that, as people age, they get more unalike one another, so it is difficult to say what is a 'normal' reaction in later life.

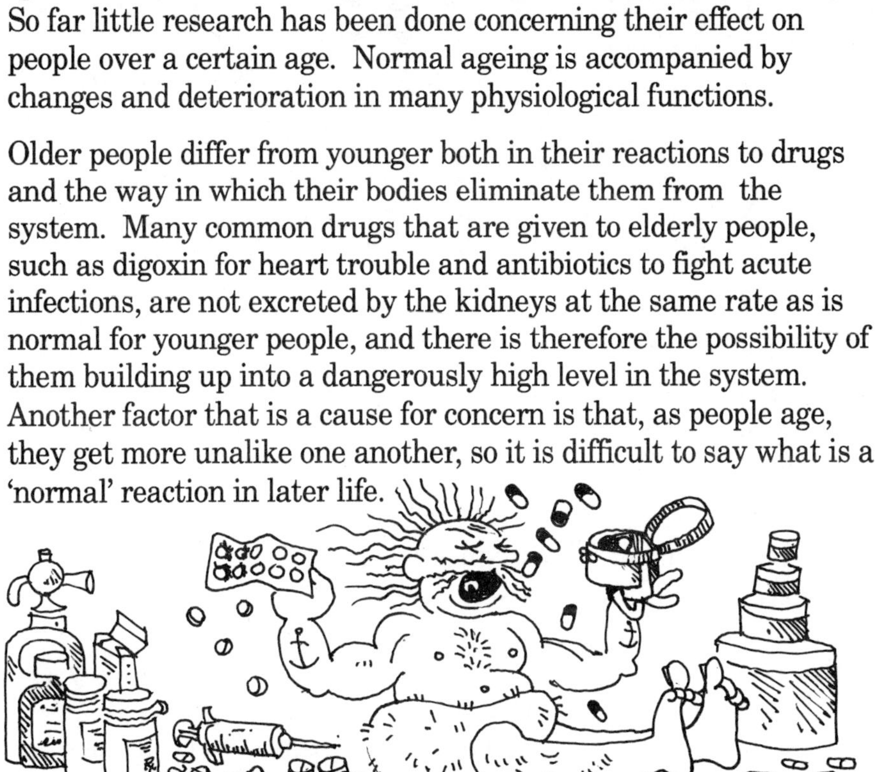

In prescribing for older people doctors must take certain risks with many drugs if they are to do any good at all, but the problem is greatly increased because with the appetite for drugs that some patients acquire they may be taking five or more drugs simultaneously. A doctor would have to be a real pharmacological wizard to know just what any complex combination of various drugs is going to do to a patient. It is no wonder that many doctors are forced to use the principle of 'suck it and see': if someone is taking five different sorts of pills and a liquid medicine, and managing to get along quite reasonably, why alter the regime? The patient may seldom see the doctor and get repeat prescriptions by applying to the reception desk.

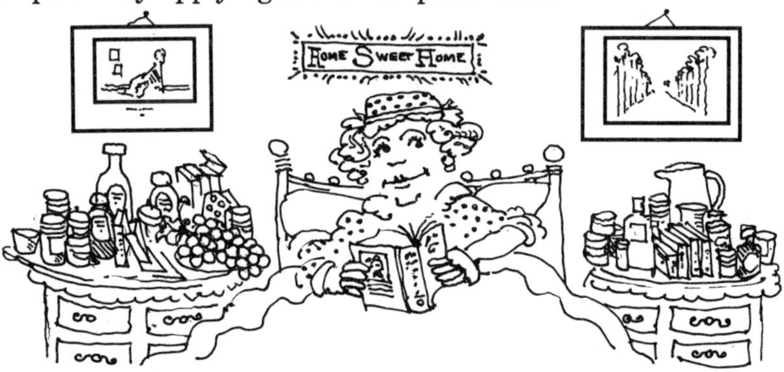

I have read of some extraordinary cases of 'polypharmacy', such as the doctor who counted 36 bottles of pills beside the bedside of a bed-ridden old lady. None of her family appeared to know what pills were for what but every few hours they gave her a few.

The question arises, how has it come about that a body of well-trained professionals who are mostly hard-working men and women of goodwill with a real humane concern for their patients have allowed this situation to develop? The answer appears to lie in the fact that the medical profession have been overtaken by a population trend that was not fully anticipated or prepared for — the great increase in the number of older people. Some doctors have not been adequately trained in the specialism of geriatric medicine and, as yet, comparatively little is known about the problems of later life. If all goes well there is little doubt that sufficient research effort will eventually elucidate these problems, but those of us in later life have simply got to accept that we are in some sense 'pioneers' in a relatively uncharted sea, and to some extent, 'guinea-pigs'. Great advances on the health front have already been made but we must be patient with our doctors.

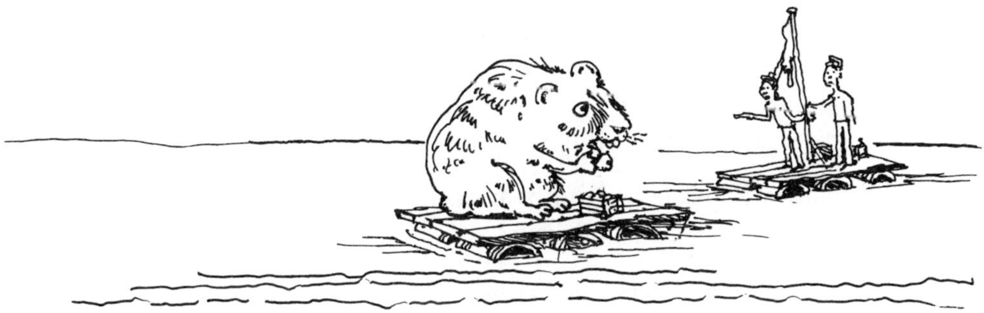

In addition to the element of uncertainty that attaches to the drug treatment of elderly people, doctors have to balance the physical effects that drugs have on their older patients against the psychological effects of issuing prescriptions. Giving a prescription helps to maintain good doctor-patient relationships in most cases, and this is essential if the latter is to be properly looked after; a doctor's reasons for giving a drug of doubtful value may sometimes be paraphrased as follows:

If I don't give him a prescription he may fuss and worry about his condition and make himself worse, whereas the condition will probably clear up of its own accord and he'll be happy taking his medicine. Also, as he appears to be a confirmed pill-swallower, if I don't give himself anything he will possibly fill himself up with unwise quantities of over-the-counter medicines and do himself real harm. On balance, I think that this is a case for another prescription, although I doubt if this drug will have any significant effect on him in the tiny quantity I am prescribing.

You may feel resentful of the idea that your doctor may be giving you drugs as a fractious child is given lollipops to calm him, but you must remember that there is a sufficient number of people in the patient population to make such a policy justified.

An editorial in *The Lancet* headed DRUGS AND THE ELDERLY gives doctors some guidelines about prescribing for elderly patients, and on the basis of this I will suggest what responsibility you, as a patient, should take, for there is little point in your doctor giving sound advice if you really have not understood what has been said — particularly if you have not told the doctor how very bad your hearing is. Consider the following points:

1. Does he / she really think you need the drug, or is the prescription merely to please you?

2. Make sure that it is clear what other drugs you are already taking.

3. Ask if the instructions for taking the medicine will be clearly printed on the label, as you might forget the verbal instructions.

4. Are you clear precisely what the medicine is supposed to do to you?

5. When this lot of medicine is finished, should you apply at the desk for a repeat prescription, or should you pay another visit to see if you should continue to take it?

6. Ask what possible side-effects might result from taking the drug, and what you should do if they occur.

7. If you remember taking this particular drug some years ago and, for instance, your face swelled up like a balloon, or you came out in purple spots, be sure to tell the doctor. It will be in your case-notes, but they may be too voluminous for anyone to read right through.

You may fear that the doctor will think that you are an old fuss-pot for asking all these questions, but at least it makes clear that you have an intelligent appreciation of all the facts associated with drug taking and that it is safe to give you the prescription – which is not always the case. Additionally, it will make sure that you are not taking a drug unnecessarily or for longer than need be.

Some doctors may not like giving you information about possible side effects, because if very suggestible patients are told that certain tablets may make their toes tingle, sure as dammit their toes will tingle even if they are given a completely dummy tablet. This unfortunate effect cannot be avoided, but as long as you are aware of it, and acquire the information about possible side-effects you will know when to stop taking the drug if serious abnormal reactions occur.

ALTERNATIVE THERAPY

The two terms 'alternative therapy' and 'complementary therapy' have come into use in modern times. The latter indicates forms of therapy in addition to what is normally supplied by medical practitioners; thus doctors may refer a patient to a qualified osteopath for special manipulative treatment of the joints if they are satisfied that this would be beneficial. People are, of course, free to take their troubles to osteopaths independently, but what these practitioners do is not inconsistent with the general medical view of human functioning. 'Alternative therapy' on the other hand, refers to treatment that is given according to systems of beliefs about human functioning which is alternative to that traditionally held in Western medicine.

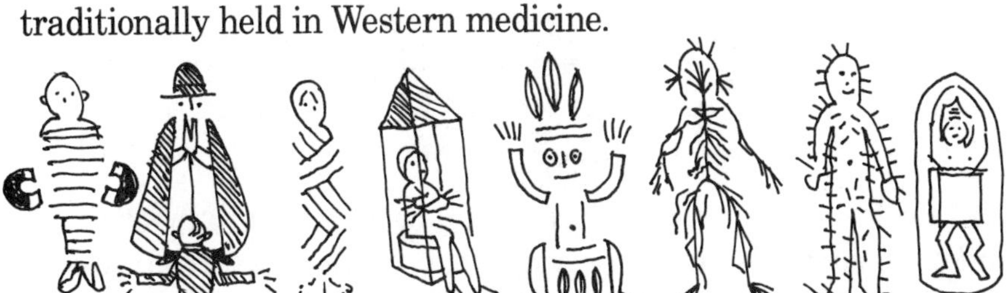

There are numerous forms of alternative therapy which have little in common with one another as to their theoretical basis, and some are quite hostile to orthodox medical practice. In 1986 the British Medical Association published a Report of their Board of Science and Education which had conducted an investigation into the more common forms of alternative therapy. In their Appendix they list 116 different forms of therapy which appear to be independent and competing with one another. Lord Skelmersdale, the Under-Secretary of Health, informed parliament during a debate on complementary therapy in November 1987, that he had identified no fewer than 160 of them.

Unconventional treatments may appeal to young people if they are in a state of rebellion against the orthodoxies of society, and hence orthodox medicine. There is something appealing about chewing ginseng when Pluto is in the house of Venus, or some other astrological twaddle, as a cure for facial acne ('Well, no-one has ever proved that it doesn't cure it, have they?') but there is a growing number of papers and magazines aimed at older and retired people, and all sorts of advertisements are appearing in them, cleverly worded so that they escape condemnation by the advertising standards authority, offering a variety of products and treatments, some obviously fraudulent, designed to cater for the health-needs of elderly people.

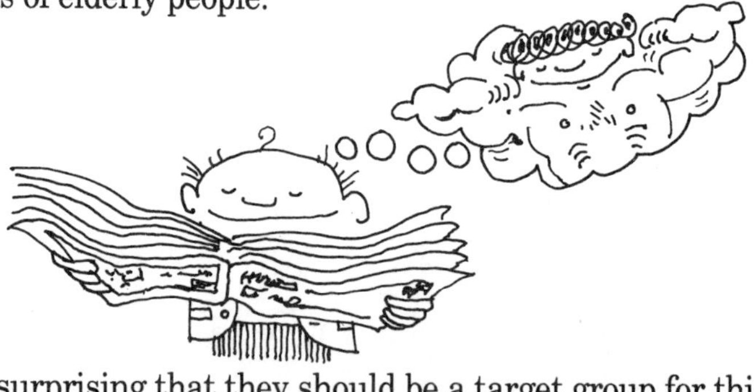

It is hardly surprising that they should be a target group for this kind of business. Many older people expect that they can lead a completely comfortable life, but later life does bring with it disabilities such as rheumatism, arthritis, heart trouble, failing sexual potency in men, osteoporosis, wrinkles, hair loss and a general failing of physical power. Orthodox medicine does not claim to be able to abolish all these ills, although there are sensible treatments that alleviate them, delay their progress, and help us to come to terms with them, but some alternative therapists claim miracles.

Consider this account of one form of alternative therapy, radionics:

> If you approach a radiesthetist, or a radionics practitioner, you will be asked to cut off some of your hair, or prick yourself with a sterilised needle and let a drop of blood fall on a piece of blotting paper. To a practitioner of radiesthesia or radionics, the hair or the blood is your 'witness'; it represents you as much as if you had presented yourself 'in person.'From it the practitioner claims to be able to ascertain your present condition, the best treatment to administer, and often any future illnesses that your body contains but has yet to manifest. This may sound far-fetched in comparison with most other alternative therapies, but radiesthesia and radionics have been practised for long enough for their shortcomings to have been exposed.

Homeopathy, the Grape Cure, iridology, naturopathy, reflexology, orgone therapy, and others have become popular precisely because they give a resounding slap in the face to common sense and the scientific approach, for some people have a strong prejudice against what they conceive to be 'science', and this includes orthodox medicine.

The alternative therapist is generally uninterested in medical diagnosis. He may start staring at the irises of the patient's eyes (iridology), or pulling his toes (reflexology) in the hope that he or she can both diagnose and treat the disorder. The defence of an alternative therapy that is often given is, that however plain foolish it sounds, it works! This is not to be denied absolutely, but in order to understand why an unorthodox system may appear to 'work', we have to consider the nature of human disease and malfunction.

The placebo response

If I were to give a number of patients suffering from disordered livers a medicine consisting of tap water coloured with some harmless plant dye, assuring them that this is a proven remedy for their condition, as long as they had faith in me as a therapist, a number of them would certainly improve, and attribute their improvement to the 'medicine' I had given them. This is known as the placebo reaction, and scientific research has shown that it can be very powerful indeed in certain circumstances and for some disorders. There is nothing very mysterious about it; it relates to the fact that all disorders have two components, an organic component and a psychological component. In certain disorders such as eczema, asthma, indigestion, migraine, the psychological factor is very large indeed, and the severity of the condition at any one time is very dependent on the patient's psychological state. This is very well known, and people are not surprised when their eczema etc. gets worse when they are worried, depressed, overworked and generally stressed. But even in conditions that are almost wholly organic, as in infective diseases, the psychological state is important in determining how effectively the body's natural defences cope with the invading agent.

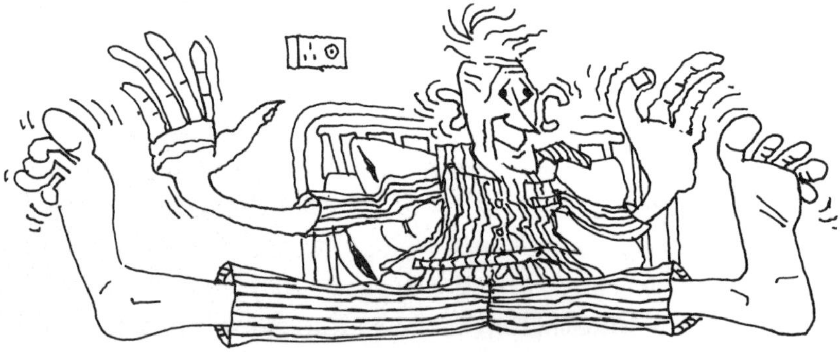

Thus, if a patient suffering from something like mumps has his toes pulled while he is told a cock-and-bull story that he is suffering from a congested spleen, providing that he believes such nonsense, and is paying a high fee to have his toes pulled ('It must be worth it – after I've paid out all that money!') he probably will feel better, and perhaps get over his mumps quicker than if he had had no such treatment.

The placebo reaction has been well known in medical research for quite a long time, and all new drugs are now tested to see if they really are more effective than an inert placebo.

In the course of any illness, even those that eventually lead to death, patients have their ups and downs, feeling better some days, or weeks, than others. This is known as the 'natural variability of disease.' Thus, practitioners of alternative therapy can run a lucrative business by capitalizing on this natural variability. It does not matter what their stock-in-trade is – it can be an elixir, a manipulative procedure, a form of posture control, an electrical hocus-pocus, a kind of psychotherapy – and it is immaterial how irrational their rationale is, provided that it is as harmless as it is useless.

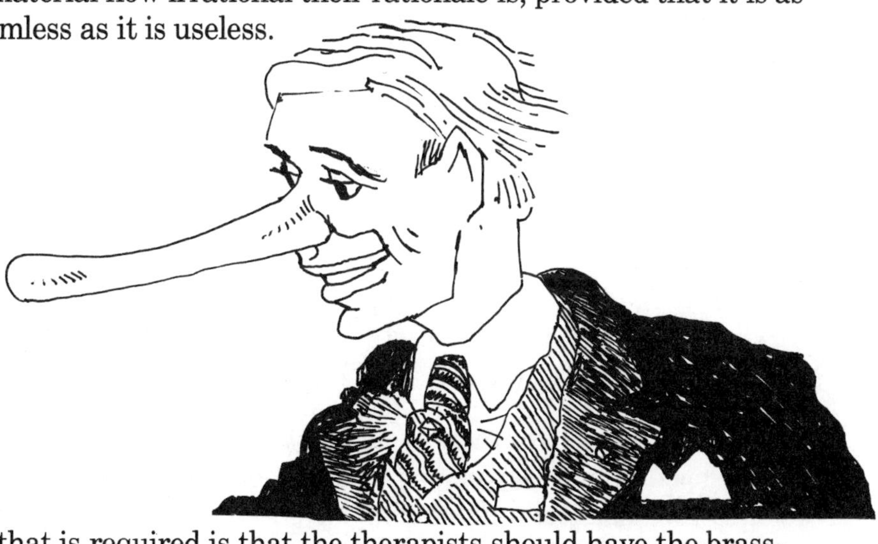

All that is required is that the therapists should have the brass-faced effrontery and smooth-talking glibness to persuade sick and gullible people to believe in it.

Ideally, for the sake of the therapist's reputation, the treatment should be first applied when the patient is at the bottom of one of his 'troughs', for the chances are that he will soon begin to feel better anyway, and the therapist can take the credit for the improvement. If however, the severity of the complaint remains the same, the patient can be persuaded that at least the treatment has checked the further deterioration that otherwise would have occurred. What is needed now is obviously more intensive treatment (and more frequent fee-paying visits). If the patient's condition continues to get even worse, it is explained that this is because he delayed too long in coming for effective treatment and it will need a really long regime of intensive alternative therapy before any improvement can be expected. If the patient then dies, the therapist need not be abashed. 'If only he had come to me sooner!' he says.

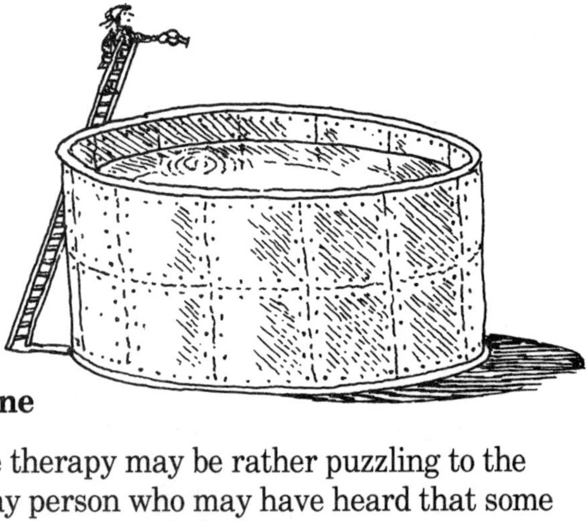

Homeopathic medicine

This view of alternative therapy may be rather puzzling to the average open-minded lay person who may have heard that some well qualified medical practitioners have in the immediate past practised 'homeopathic medicine' (and some perhaps still do). This was discussed in the BMA Report, which explained how in the late 18th century doctors were using harmful drugs, often in prodigious doses, to the detriment of their patients who sometimes died under such treatment. Samuel Hahnemann developed the theory that drugs which gave rise to the symptoms of a disease could be used to combat that disease. Thus cinchola bark produces a fever like that indicative of malaria when administered in a strong enough dose, but its extract, quinine, is an effective remedy in treating malaria. Hahnemann's experiments led him to administer drugs in absolutely minute quantities dissolved in water, and later he incorporated into his homeopathic theory certain mystical ideas of 'vitalism'. He came to believe that the enormously diluted solutions that he administered served to act upon the patients' 'vital force' and so bring about healing.

Obviously in the late 18th and early 19th centuries the homeopathic doctors who followed Hahnemann and administered only tremendously diluted solutions of drugs had better success than their medical colleagues who often gave their patients harmful drugs in rather large quantities because pharmacology was then in its infancy. The mystical and wholly irrational element of homeopathy continues today, and the BMA Report sets out to answer the following question:

> What then is the explanation of the survival of homeopathy . . . essentially in the form devised by its founder, by which alkali or metallic salts, the metals themselves or their oxides, or the more toxic of the then used simples are prescribed, usually in solutions so great, and in doses so minute as to have no pharmacological action, and sometimes in dilutions that are unlikely to contain a single surviving molecule?

They point out that the homeopathic practitioner believes in the existence of an 'immaterial force' residing in the medicines that are prescribed, and patients are induced to believe in this also, and thus 'it appears that, a placebo effect is the explanation of the belief, shared by homeopaths and their patients, in the efficacy of homeopathic therapeutics.'

The European Commission proposes rules for the registration of medicines in the associated countries, and very extensive and conclusive proof of their effectiveness has to be given. These measures produced a panic among companies who had been manufacturing drugs for many years – including the homeopaths. A medical advisor to the Belgian Ministry of Health, Dr Wim Betz, was called upon to give advice about the validity of homeopathic medicine and he writes:

> Other protesters were the homeopathy adepts who for obvious reasons would face big problems meeting these demands of proven efficiency. They have lobbied for these directives to be adapted to the special properties of homeopathic medicines (HM) and Anthroposophic Medicine (AM) so as to dispense them from their burden of scientific proof.

As the Belgian Ministry of Health seemed reluctant to accept his recommendations regarding the uselessness of homeopathy, he demanded that all forms of 'alternative therapy', including the most ludicrous, should receive equal recognition, and added:

> It should be all or none. If any serious progress is made on the path to recognition of some therapies with the exclusion of others we must officially and vehemently protest the violation of our right to free choice. I, for myself, intend to demand that gemmotherapy and oenotherapy (treatment by precious stones and good wine) be made available to me, all expenses paid on the national health.

THE ANTI-SCIENCE ATTITUDE

Many older people have a strong wish to believe in the nonscientific, the irrational. They live in a technological culture and feel constantly menaced by the dangers around them that they attribute to scientific advancement. Their belief-systems are based on some truths, half-truths and even sometimes, downright nonsense. As they perceive it, we now live in a ruined world: the atmosphere is being polluted by the exhausts of motor cars; the crops are being sprayed with harmful pesticides; electricity may be emanating from the power-lines and even, perhaps, domestic power-sockets, ruining our health; radio-activity leaks out of smoke-detectors and clobbers us; fluoride salts and other poisons are added to our drinking-water by mad scientists; doctors menace our health with drugs and 'unnatural' procedures.

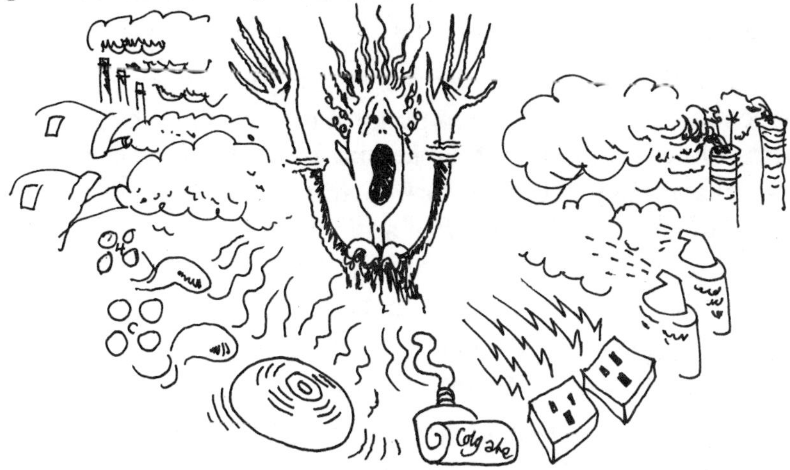

Many older people are prey to such fears and look nostalgically back at 'the good old days' when things were simpler. Such people ignore the obvious facts about the vast improvements in public health during the present century in the more developed countries that have virtually wiped out many of the infective epidemics and greatly increased the expectation of life. To them 'scientists' are still the villains who menace us all, and scientifically based medicine is highly suspect. They would much rather go to therapists who promise them 'natural' cures that do not stand up to any kind of rational examination.

THE DOCTORS' RESPONSE TO ALTERNATIVE THERAPY

The medical profession is still in the process of recovering from a past in which they were too authoritarian and covered up their ignorance, and consciousness of having made many really serious mistakes, by a pretence of omnipotence. Now that they are more truly scientific in their procedures they are prepared to be more honest with the lay public. With regard to alternative therapy many doctors wish to show how open-minded they are and concerned not to be seen as condemning all unorthodox practices out of hand.

At the practice I attend there are a number of folders in the waiting-room giving patients all manner of information about various health services that are available, and I found among them a file giving information about the local Acupuncture Clinic, where none of the staff is medically qualified and which takes patients without any medical referral. It also gives some general information about acupuncture, including the fact that some properly qualified doctors in this country are using acupuncture, and are prepared to train colleagues in the practice.

In 1986 the British Medical Association published a Report on Alternative Therapy which contains a section on acupuncture which begins by pointing out:

> An alternative therapy that has captured the imagination of the public and the [medical] profession is acupuncture, the ancient Chinese art of healing. It has been in use in Europe also for two hundred and fifty years, though its popularity here, as in China, has fluctuated through the ages.

The Report goes on to point out that the current practice of acupuncture takes two forms: that which adheres to the principles of traditional Chinese medicine, and a modified form that has been adopted by doctors trained in Western medicine and which is mainly concerned with the treatment of painful conditions. Some doctors writing in *The Lancet* have been very scornful of the use of acupuncture by Western medical practitioners, but most GPs preserve a neutral stance, and the BMA Report gives a very fair account of the nature and history of acupuncture in the West.

Dr Felix Mann became prominent in the UK for his advocacy of acupuncture and ran courses in it, but after two decades disillusion set in, and Dr Mann was forced to admit that he had been rather over-optimistic. In 1979 he wrote:

> Acupuncture anaesthesia (really analgesia) works only, in my experience (though others who are experts disagree) in the hyper-strong reactor. In 1974 I reported the results of a hundred experiments in acupuncture analgesia and came to the conclusion that it worked reasonably, though not perfectly, in 10% of patients. Since then I have come to the conclusion that the criteria I used were a little optimistic, and the figure should be revised to a mere 5%.

What is the truth of the matter? I shall attempt, as a nonmedical man, to sum up the attitude of a sceptical doctor who permits, even encourages, the odd patient to try acupuncture and other forms of alternative therapy for his ill-defined disorders:

The public at large have all sorts of strange ideas about health, and there is really nothing much we doctors can do about it. They come to us expecting miracles and refusing to accept the plain fact that we don't know what's wrong with a lot of them, especially the more elderly patients, and probably never will know, for many of their ills are engendered by their imagination, and the unfortunate way in which they conduct their lives. We would like to operate within the bounds of rational medicine, but they demand that we act as shamans and priests.

Medicine has done wonders for the population at large, but they want the impossible – always to be free of all pain and sickness. A lot of patients privately sneer at the limitations of conventional medicine and want something better, for they have read about the wonders of alternative therapy in some magazine. Well, if they want acupuncture and other forms of unconventional therapy, let them have it. Some doctors do indeed believe in a limited form of acupuncture, and it appears to work with some disorders. Medically qualified acupuncturists will be better able to diagnose when patients are really suffering from some recognizable disease, and not try needling them for entirely inappropriate conditions as some lay practitioners may do. But if we try to reserve acupuncture only for medically qualified professionals then we will be accused of pursuing restrictive practices, selfishly trying to discourage patients from receiving the benefits that alternative therapists may provide.

Perhaps a middle course is better – if asked, to inform our patients about the nature of acupuncture and other popular forms of alternative therapy and leave it to them to decide what course to follow, while we will simply get on with our proper job of promoting the health of those we can help according to the tenets of scientific medicine.

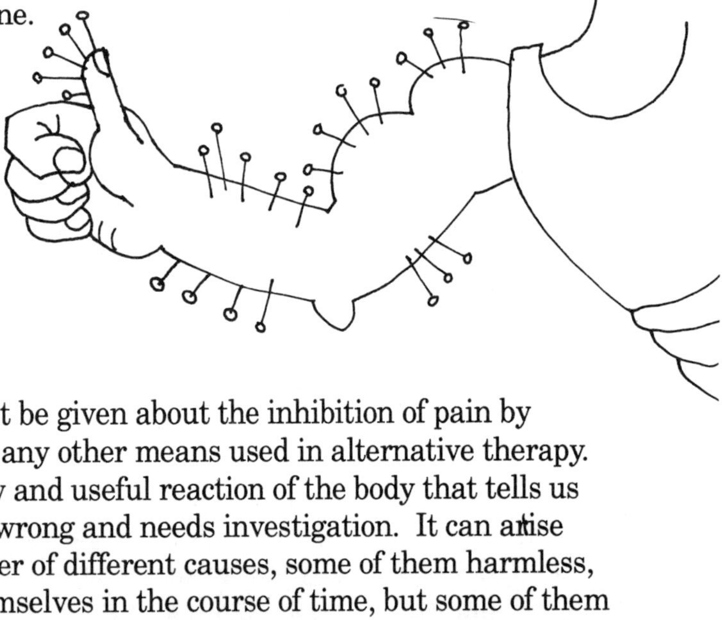

A final caveat must be given about the inhibition of pain by acupuncture or by any other means used in alternative therapy. Pain is a necessary and useful reaction of the body that tells us that something is wrong and needs investigation. It can arise from a huge number of different causes, some of them harmless, that will right themselves in the course of time, but some of them indicating the beginnings of a disease process that may be serious if left unchecked. It is foolish simply to inhibit the experience of pain without knowing what is causing it, and the investigation of painful conditions may involve x-rays, blood tests and other technical means that are more available in modern medicine.

THE DOCTORS' DILEMMA WITH OLDER PATIENTS

The doctor's dilemma consists essentially of trying to avoid falling into the trap of, on the one hand, conducting potentially damaging and unnecessary over-investigation of an elderly patient, having failed to realize that the marked difference between conventionally 'normal' results (which are accepted and taught in medical schools), and those obtained from elderly people and, on the other hand, the doctor may assume that the elderly patient's complaints are just due to his age, when in reality immediate treatment is needed. The signs of illness change with age; some disorders such as pneumonia would put you in a high fever in middle-age, but when you are older the temperature may not rise initially but the infection may result in a sort of mental confusion. Consequently some older people who have contracted pneumonia have been regarded as 'head cases' and put into the care of psychiatrists, when all that was needed was a course of antibiotics to get rid of the infection and they would have returned to normal.

It might seem that I am suggesting that you should study to be a specialist in geriatric medicine and go in for self-treatment, but I certainly do not advocate this. All that I am advising is that you should continue to take responsibility for yourself and, in doing so, realize that what went for you when you were younger will not necessarily apply in later life.

You cannot always depend on measuring yourself against friends and family who are the same age as you, for the age-marker is deceptive. In your relations with doctors and other health-care professionals, you should fully appreciate the nature of the dilemmas that they face. Earlier I referred to two extreme stereotypes of relations between doctors and patients, but I think that we are approaching a better working relationship. Geriatrics, as a special-ity within medicine, is relatively new and rapidly developing.

YOUR FINAL RESPONSIBILITY

As with all professions – solicitors, architects, accountants, dentists – you may chance to be just unlucky, and it is up to you, having appreciated all the difficulties under which doctors must work, to exercise your right of choice. Dr Alex Comfort, who has little patience with his more backward medical colleagues, gives this advice:

> Fly like the plague from the kind of veterinary technician who thinks anyone over seventy is likely (without further cause) suddenly to become senile or crazy, who tells you to 'expect' illness, in terms of passive contemplation, as a normal state of older people, or who dislikes the old. If you were a dog he'd have you put down. Such doctors are now fortunately getting rarer.

A woman who has nursed an arthritic hip for ten years obviously does not know as much about arthritis as her doctor does, but she may be an expert on her hip and how it should be managed – never mind what the medical textbook says – and an intelligent doctor will recognize this. Do not reject or despise advice from properly trained health-care professionals but remember that the responsibility for your health lies with yourself. Happily, 'a little of what you fancy does you good', but you should make informed choices and guide your fancy on the basis of knowledge, and not according to old wives' tales, or the latest 'health' magazine bought on a railway bookstall.

Chapter 7

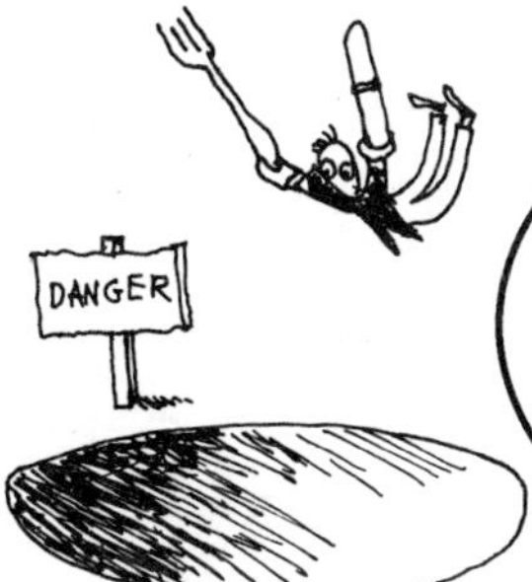

SOME PITFALLS IN LATER LIFE

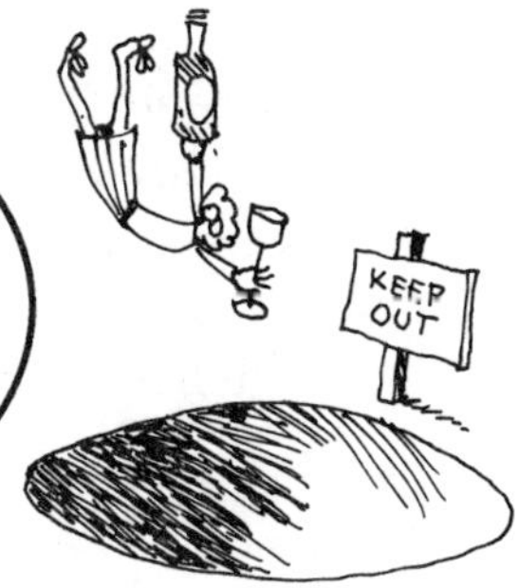

Some activities and habits that are necessary and relatively harmless for most of our lives, bear certain risks when we are in the Third Age and may lead to ill-health and perhaps an early demise. You should examine the more common of them and consider what changes you may wish to make in your life-style.

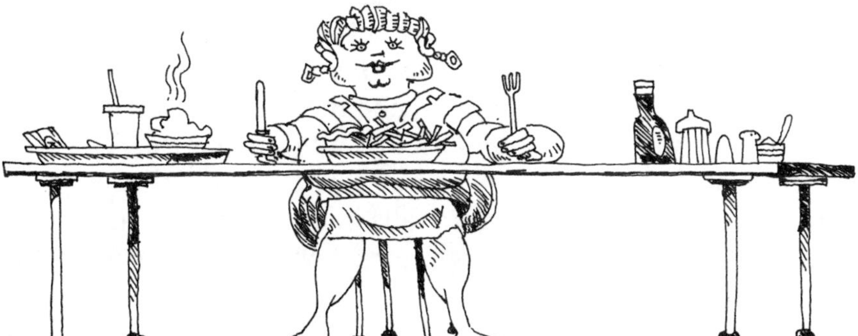

EATING

I sometimes go to a university canteen, and I see there a lady who is probably in her late 30s and is quite remarkably fat. I see her going to a table bearing a tray loaded with a really solid meal. She likes food such as a steak and kidney pie with chips, followed by a steamed pudding with custard, and I have sometimes observed a bar of chocolate on the tray, possibly to be consumed during the afternoon. She sits there eating this meal among all those skinny girl students pecking at their salads and brown rolls; she seems as happy as can be, as she overflows an inadequate plastic chair that looks silly under her great bulk. With her ruddy fat cheeks and glossy hair she looks the picture of health, and perhaps she is very healthy, but alas, what lies ahead of her in later life if she continues to be so massively fat?

In later life over-eating and consequent fatness carries certain grave risks. Fat people are liable to develop a diabetic tendency when they are older, and diabetes of Type II is a disease that may have various serious consequences. The excess glucose in the blood produces degenerative changes in the nerves, blood vessels, kidneys and retina. Heart disease and impotence in the male are among the consequences of diabetes.

Apart from diabetes there are other purely mechanical risks arising from being greatly over-weight in later life. Earlier in life the muscles and bones may be strong enough to support a huge burden of fat, but there is an inevitable decline in muscular strength with ageing and it may become just too much effort to take a proper amount of exercise, and the over-fat individual then suffers from various disorders that result from inertia . The excess weight may do damage to the joints, particularly to the hip joints and knees. Broken bones due to falls in later life are a not uncommon danger, and an over-weight person will sustain more damage from a fall.

Food can be a great pleasure, and perhaps it was better appreciated in the last century. We seem a little ashamed of it today and the cult of dieting and slimness has been fashionable for half a century. We can look back to a time when it was a matter for congratulation that:

Augustus was a chubby lad;

Fat ruddy cheeks Augustus had:

And everybody saw with joy,

The plump and hearty, healthy boy.

But while you should still have a keen and healthy appreciation of the pleasures of the table, and bear in mind that some of us were born to be fat, and others to be thin, it is as well to realize that in later life you may 'dig your grave with your teeth'. You should therefore learn to enjoy your food for its quality rather than its quantity, and to stay healthy in later life you need to take the trouble to plan your meals so that you really do enjoy them. Once you have understood the simple facts of diet, as set out in Chapter 4, then a little of what you fancy will indeed do you good.

WHAT IS A NORMAL WEIGHT?

You may wonder what is a 'normal' weight for your height, age and sex. Statistics based on thousands of men and women have been worked out and published in tables. The ratio of weight to height is known as the Body Mass Index (BMI) and is calculated in metric measurements and obtained by the formula:

(Weight in kg) divided by (height in metres squared)

(kg / m^2). The following guidelines are given:

BMI below 20.0 = underweight.

BMI above 25.0 = overweight.

BMI above 30.0 = obesity.

Thus if a woman in her early 60s is 5ft 4ins in height, a weight anywhere between 8 stone 5 lbs and 10 stone 6 lbs is within the normal range; anything over the higher limit can be regarded as 'overweight', and if she is over 12 stone 7lbs she is 'obese'. It does not matter in later life if you are a little overweight; it is more a cause for worry if you are seriously underweight, and unfortunate consequences may follow from being too thin, as will be explained later.

If you wish to work out your own BMI as a matter of interest, remember to convert your weight to kilograms and your height to metres.

The dangers of food-poisoning

Alas that such a delightful thing as food should threaten our health and even our lives increasingly as we get older. The plain fact is that older people are more vulnerable to the special sorts of bacteria that may contaminate food. When you were younger you could cope with just a tiny dose of listeria, salmonella, campylobacter and other nasty creatures. You may have had a little tummy upset and felt out of sorts for a bit, but now you are older you may be seriously ill if they attack you. The following are the main risks of food-poisoning, and some suggestions for avoiding them:

1. You are reluctant to waste food and hence hoard leftovers, sometimes reheating them before you consume them. This is especially true if you are hard up and live on your own. Don't! Grit your teeth and throw the leftovers away unless they are simple things like cold potatoes that are immediately put in the fridge.

2. Some foods are particularly liable to be contaminated, such as eggs, liver patés, and soft cheeses. Although you may love soft boiled eggs, it is safer to cook them properly. Be wary about the uncooked food you buy.

3. Frozen foods may look and smell all right but they may harbour some nasty bacteria. See that you unfreeze them thoroughly before you cook them, because live organisms may still lurk in the middle that has not been thoroughly cooked.

4. If dangerous bacteria are present in what you buy they will continue to breed as long as you keep the food. Therefore see that your fridge is working properly and is not just a damp cupboard, and do not eat food after the sell-by date that is printed on the package. Throw it away!

5. When you were younger you used to eat at Joe's cafe where the food was cheap but the plates were smeary. Now you are older consider the fact that a lot of food-poisoning is caused by the handling and preparation of food in unhygienic conditions. Even though you may be very hard up, do be careful where you eat and what you eat there. While a robust young lorry-driver may eat a dubious fish pie and get away with it, you may not be so lucky.

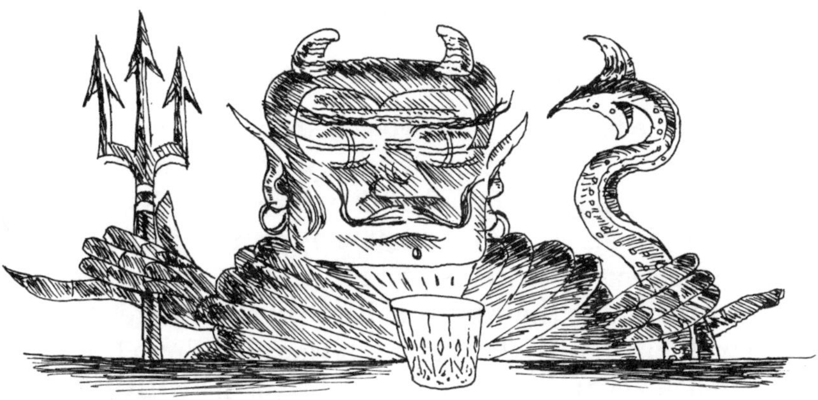

DRINKING

Giving guidance regarding drinking alcoholic liquor is very difficult. All books giving advice on health in later life have something to say about this subject but there is little agreement between the 'experts'. The subject of drinking seems to activate views that are often influenced by their degree of moralism that does not shape their other opinions about health matters. We are all agreed that alcohol is and has always been widely abused in our society and can be a cause of a great deal of ill-health, personal and social misery, and society therefore has a sort of love-hate relationship with it, while many Muslim countries outlaw its use entirely. In Christian countries there has always been a vociferous 'temperance' movement which veers between wishing to exclude alcoholic drinks entirely from our usage, and urging us to drink only 'in moderation'. But what on earth does moderation mean?

Many people in later life who wish to enjoy their remaining years to the full may justifiably resent over-cautious advice from younger people who lean too heavily towards a temperance attitude in advising their elders, and appreciate Edward Fitzgerald's advice:

Come, fill the cup and in the fire of Spring,

The winter garment of repentance fling:

The bird of time has but a little way

To fly — and Lo! The bird is on the wing.

Maybe it would be better for you if you drank only carrot juice, but when 'The bird is on the wing' you may reflect that what is important is the quality of life rather than its length. Regarding the carrot juice, I once read an account of a coroner's inquest on a cranky man who was so concerned for his health that he appears to have lived mainly on the stuff, and hence died of carotene poisoning with his skin bright yellow! If you suffer from heart trouble, and many of us in the Third Age do, you may have been cheered by some recent medical research of Cambridge scientists which showed that red wine was of positive benefit to the heart, and that moderate wine-bibbers lived longer than abstainers. I think it must have been this research that impelled a medical writer on health in later life to say:

> Alcohol . . . in moderate quantities, is quite good for you. Any man will live longer for taking six glasses of wine a day, a woman three glasses, rather than remaining abstemious.

But this doctor is referring to six glasses of wine a day as being described as being 'in moderate quantities'. Have we got here the actual definition of 'moderation' that we all crave for? Yet elsewhere in the same book this writer prescribes as a maximum amount of daily intake: '. . . approximately two bottles of beer, or three glasses of wine or two cocktails.' Here is a typical example of the vagueness in which some 'experts' like to clothe their advice about our drinking alcohol. They prompt one to ask – how big is a bottle of beer and how strong is the wine? At my local off-licence the bottles of beer vary much in size and strength, and the proof of the common wines are from 9% to 13%. Amongst the 'experts' who are more puritanical about alcohol and like to make our flesh creep, one writes:

'. . . basically, as at any age – if you find you cannot do without alcohol you should drop it entirely, with professional help if need be. The average time it takes to convince an alcoholic that he or she has a medical problem is fifteen years, and in old age you don't have that long. Also, as at earlier ages, drinking is often a covert form of suicide.'

Isn't that enough to put the wind up you? But perhaps the words 'cannot do without alcohol' introduce a certain vagueness, and many of us will wonder whether or not we could do without the stuff if we tried, but we don't intend to make the experiment. Your thoughts may turn to many famous figures who never tried to find out whether they could totally abstain. Sir Winston Churchill, who lived to the age of 91 and was remarkably active in his old age, was apparently never worried on this score. The tales of his boisterousness in his cups are legion, and when once reproved by a lady member of the House: "Winston – you are drunk!" he was moved to reply most rudely: "And you, Madam, are ugly. But I'll be sober tomorrow!"

Here you may well ask – 'Is there no scientific evidence on the subject, and should it not be included in such a book as this?'

DANGERS OF THE DEMON DRINK

While perhaps sympathising with the positive view of wine that the poet Edward Fitzgerald put forward (his poem was supposed to be a very free translation from the Persian *The Rubiayat of Omar Kayyam*), in order to enjoy drink and benefit from it, you should be fully aware of its dangers. According to a report of the World Health Organization (WHO), 5 to 12% of men, and 1 to 2% of women in their 60s are 'problem drinkers'. If you were to ask most retired people whether they have any problem with drink, they would probably reply 'Yes – it's too expensive!' but what the WHO means is that those people are damaging their health by drinking more than is good for them.

Unlike most of the writers who vaguely caution you to be 'moderate' in your drinking, the WHO gives some useful facts and figures about alcoholic drinks. They measure alcohol in units irrespective of the drink that contains it: a single unit equals half a pint of beer, or one glass of wine, or a small sherry, or a single measure of spirits. The following table shows the weekly consumption of alcohol in terms of units in relation to the risk-category of the drinker – that is, the risk of their becoming a 'problem drinker'.

RISK	WOMEN	MEN
Low	up to 14 units	up to 21
Moderate	15 - 35	22 - 49
High	36 +	50 +

It will be observed that the average man may safely drink more than the average woman. Thus he may drink in a week up to 21 units ($10\frac{1}{2}$ pints of beer) and still be in the low-risk category, but she must limit her drinking to only 14 units (7 pints of beer). This sounds like a most unfair sexist judgement, but don't be misled by it. The fact is that it refers to averages; the average man is bigger and heavier than the average woman, and the bigger the bulk of the body the more alcohol it can tolerate. While I was working in Japan I noticed that Japanese people got drunk quicker and with less drink than their European companions, and realized that this was largely due to the fact that the Japanese are smaller on average. So, as the physiology of women is just the same as that of men with regard to alcohol, a big woman with a small husband may safely out-match him at the bar.

Good news for older drinkers.

Recent medical research has shown that light to moderate intake of alcohol is of positive advantage to the continued health of older people. It reduces the risk of coronary heart disease by as much as 50%, and it also reduces their susceptibility to one form of stroke - 'ischaemic stroke'. The latter term refers to damage to the brain when the supply of oxygen is drastically reduced because the arteries become narrowed.

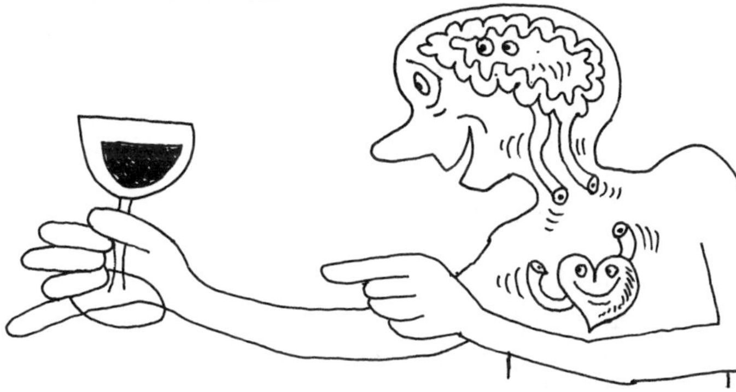

It is ironic that this benefit is specially conferred on older people rather than young and middle-aged people, for you may be accustomed to the pundits telling you that you should be more and more cautious in your habits as you get older. The reason for this paradox is that for many substances that bring positive benefits there is also a negative risk to be considered. Alcohol does no good at all to the liver, and the risk of breast and bowel cancer may be increased, as does the risk of 'haemorrhagic stroke' – brain damage due to breaking of blood-vessels in the brain – so you must watch it! The fact is that the chances of coronary disease and ischaemic stroke are not very great in the earlier part of your life, so younger people do not get much benefit from drinking alcohol, but later on when the risk is greater it is certainly worth while considering the advantages of moderate drinking. In France the incidence of coronary heart disease is remarkably low, and it is likely that this is related to the French habit of drinking wine at mealtimes as a matter of course.

With many things you have to consider the balance of benefits and disadvantages, and these alter as you get older. With the life-style of young and middle-aged people drinking all too often has disastrous consequences, and this is not only through damaging their health by over-stepping the weekly limit as defined above. Two or three extra beers with the boys at a party, and then a fast dash home in the car so as not to incur too much wrath from the wife, or rushing off to a better party, has frequently been the cause of death and injury to themselves as well as others, but as oldies tend not to have that sort of life-style they are less exposed to that sort of risk. Other risks in later life have to be considered.

Psychological addiction

Alcohol is not an addictive drug in the same sense that, say, opium is. The opium eater has to take more and more of his drug as time goes on in order to get the same effect, but those who drink alcoholic drinks will continue to get the same result for the same amount of tipple without needing to increase it. Psychological addiction is another matter; thus if someone is accustomed to drink seven pints of beer with his mates every Saturday night, he will feel seriously unhappy if they all decide to go on the wagon and expect him to be content with lemonade. Again, if someone is accustomed to hit the bottle when any crisis arrives in their lives (their spouse threatens to leave them, they are in danger of eviction, the bank manager finally loses patience . . .) if alcohol is unavailable they will indeed be in a tizzy. Some people try to cope with the difficulties that may occur in later life – loneliness, ill-health, money worries, painful conditions like arthritis – by resort to alcohol. This is all very well in the short run; why shouldn't you use whisky when the doctor's drugs for your painful back seem pretty useless? But this is dangerous if it becomes a psychological addiction. To wrestle with the ills of later life, just as with the problems that challenge us at any age, we need to brace ourselves to do something active about them, and just retiring into an alcoholic haze will certainly not help.

It is certainly not clear whether people in later life drink more heavily than younger people. The latter tend to drink more socially, and may encourage each other to consume more than is good for them, but the danger is that older people, especially if they live on their own, may go in for solitary drinking. If those on a pension are hard up, there is a danger that they may spend money on drink that should be better spent on nourishing food, and this will do them no good at all. If you are going to drink rather heavily for a period you should certainly eat properly.

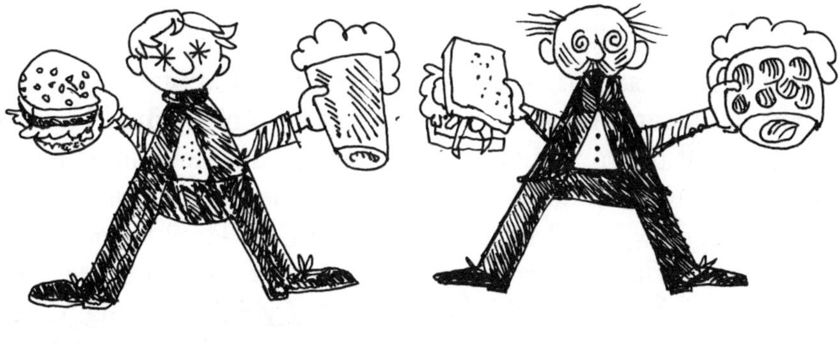

The remedy for drinking too much is not the attempted cultivation of 'an iron will' and making repeated resolutions to say 'No!', as such resolutions are generally very soluble in alcohol. The common-sense remedy lies in taking active steps to try to overcome the causes of the malaise that drives you to drink. Membership of a group such as Alcoholics Anonymous can be very helpful indeed if you are really an extreme case of alcoholism, not so much because of the stated ideology and religious commitment of AA, but because once the alcoholic is enmeshed in a closely supportive group, he or she will no longer be lonesome and forlorn, and hence has less need to tipple.

Finally, having given some facts and figures culled from the WHO report, let me make a most important observation: it has been pointed out that in later life people may be very different from one another. There are enormous variations in their individual reactions to alcohol, both physically and mentally. Earlier I mentioned Sir Winston Churchill and his liberal drinking; I am sure that if I consumed his weekly amount of alcohol I would be knocked sideways. Similarly, if a teetotaller suddenly began to drink even my modest intake of alcohol he would be quite upset. So what do you do in later life if you want guidance as to what is a 'moderate' intake of alcohol?

The figures given by the WHO may be of some use, but they must be interpreted in view of what has suited you best in the past. Some 'experts' say that tolerance of alcohol decreases with age, but this is more an opinion than a fact based upon actual research. Perhaps it is true for some people but not for others, and I have a suspicion that tolerance may even increase. You alone must be the final arbiter in this matter as in so many others.

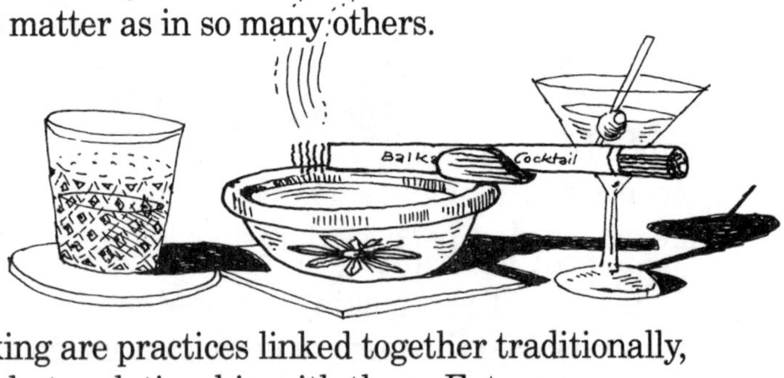

SMOKING

Smoking and drinking are practices linked together traditionally, and we have a love-hate relationship with them. Extreme moralists have lumped them together and condemned them (together with sex), as in the temperance song:

Cigarettes and whiskey, and wild, wild women –

They drive a man crazy, they drive him insane!

The same song describes the cigarette as having 'A fool at one end and a fire at the other'. Because of the present-day campaign against smoking, many places of public use and entertainment ban the practice, and one of the last bastions of the smoker is the public house, because drinkers smoke and smokers drink. Really, however, there is not a great similarity between alcohol and tobacco smoke; the former is a depressant drug which, by depressing the 'higher centres of control' may make you merry and relaxed, whereas the latter contains a stimulant drug, nicotine, which peps you up and has the effect of 'steadying the nerves'. Alcohol is not really an addictive drug in a physical sense, but nicotine is, and you may suffer withdrawal symptoms whilst giving up smoking.

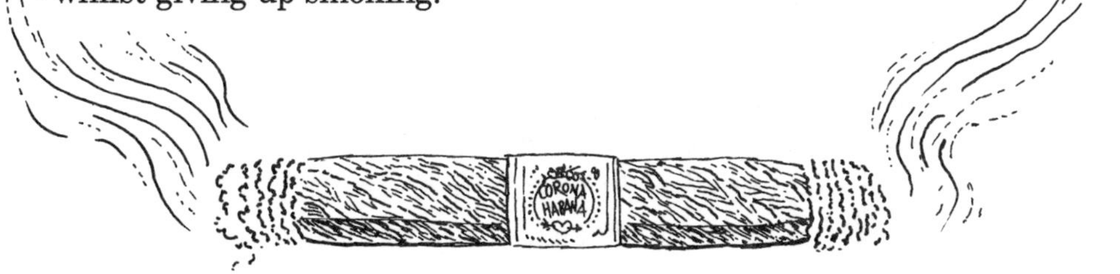

Both habits lend themselves to psychological addiction, however, and experts are divided as to the relative proportions of physiological and psychological addiction that account for the difficulty many people have in breaking the smoking habit. While moderate drinking has now been shown to be beneficial in later life, no-one now believes that smoking is of positive benefit to health.

It is ironic that the medical profession are now unanimously agreed that smoking is a wholly harmful thing, whereas it used to be held that tobacco in its many forms was medically beneficial to health. Many panegyrics in praise of 'the tawny weed' may be quoted. Byron praised tobacco as being:

Divine in hookahs, glorious in a pipe,

When tipp'd with amber, mellow, rich and ripe;

Like other charmers, wooing the caress

More dazzling when daring in full dress;

Yet thy true lovers admire by far

Thy naked beauties — give me a cigar!

Robert Burton in his *Anatomy of Melancholy* is full of praise for: 'Tobacco, divine, rare, superexcellent tobacco, which goes all beyond their panaceas, potable gold and philosophers' stones, a sovereign remedy for all diseases.' This was indeed the general opinion in the 17th century and beyond, but Burton also saw the negative side of the 'beneficent' weed, for he also wrote something about tobacco that has a more modern ring:

> But, as it is commonly abused by most men, which take it as tinkers do ale, 'tis a plague, a mischief, a violent purger of goods, lands, health, hellish, devilish, and damned tobacco, the ruin and overthrow of body and soul.

The medical argument

The campaign against smoking did not begin seriously until the 1950s. Up until then it was generally recognized that smoking might exacerbate lung troubles of various kinds, and doctors advised patients to give up or cut down their smoking when they complained of bronchitis, coughs, wheezing and similar troubles. It was when statisticians demonstrated that there was a definite association between smoking and the incidence of both lung cancer and heart attacks that the British Medical Association decided to launch a campaign aimed at eliminating the smoking habit altogether. But it is one thing to tell the public to give up smoking, and to discourage children from ever taking it up, and another to succeed in getting them to do so. There will always be those who are reluctant to believe ill of their loved-one and advance common-sense arguments such as 'Well my old dad smoked like a chimney and he was hale and hearty right up until his nineties!'

It is noteworthy that the government health warning printed on cigarette packets does not tell you that smoking *will* seriously damage your health, but that it *may*. The fact is that because two things are frequently found together, like smoking and lung cancer, the former does not necessarily cause the latter. It is conceivable that some people with irritable lungs and are prone to develop lung cancer, find tobacco smoke very soothing and therefore smoke heavily. Various eminent statisticians in the 1960s and 1970s claimed that the available evidence did not justify the conclusion that smoking causes lung cancer, and that the official medical argument was much too simplistic.

Certainly it must be admitted that the matter is very complex and factors other than smoking, especially a genetic predisposition, appear to contribute to the development of lung cancer in later life. It has been pointed out that lung cancer is 30% more likely to develop in the 10% of individuals who have a particular genetic make-up. Psychologist, Hans Eysenck, who was always one to embroil himself in controversial issues, made the point that:

> Even if we were to take the correlation between smoking and lung cancer seriously as a proof of causal connections, we would still have to conclude that smoking was neither a necessary nor a sufficient cause. Roughly speaking, only one heavy smoker in ten dies of lung cancer, thus smoking is not a sufficient cause. One person in ten of those who die of lung cancer is a non-smoker, thus smoking is not a necessary cause.

I am certainly not trying to argue in favour of smoking, for I am perfectly sure that the great majority of smokers would be healthier if they kicked the habit, and not just because of its association with lung cancer and heart disease. All sorts of troubles may be exacerbated by smoking; it is not just the tar getting into the lungs and the nicotine into the system, for tobacco smoke contains all sorts of deleterious chemicals, such as carbon monoxide, that can have harmful effects.

My position is that it is better to be safe than sorry. You may be one of those rare individuals who are genetically predisposed to be resistant to the harmful effects of tobacco smoke, but you may seriously damage your health or kill yourself in the process of investigating whether you are or not. However, in this book I aim to address you as a responsible adult who is to be trusted to balance risks and benefits, and to look after your health in a reasonable manner when you know the facts, rather than trying to frighten you into 'doing as doctor says', which is the line taken in some books on health. If people know the facts they are more likely to follow the advice that has emerged from modern research.

Giving up smoking

It is now widely accepted that giving up smoking at *any age* is beneficial. If you decide to quit, what do you do about it? This is a difficult question, and the answer may lie in why you smoke. If you ask two people why they smoke, one may say, 'Because I like it of course!', but the other may reply 'Because every time I try to give it up I feel so irritable and wretched that I have to have a cigarette!' The former type of people may have little difficulty in stopping smoking if they want to; they may measure the pleasure they get from smoking against the harm it may do, or is doing, to their health and decide to take the prudent course of abstinence. The latter type is in trouble however; they are addicted for both physiological and psychological reasons, and have to struggle, seeking help from the various sources that offer it.

At the surgery of the medical practice I attend there is a folder devoted to 'cures' for the smoking habit, and there are no less than twelve different pamphlets in it. Why so many? The fact is that the 'experts' are not agreed about the reasons why people smoke and what they can do about it. Many of these 'cures' assume that there is just one reason why people are addicted to tobacco, and one way to get rid of the addiction. A more reasonable approach recognizes that there are many, many different reasons why you may smoke and have difficulty in abandoning the habit. It would be idle for me to recommend one 'cure' rather than another.

If you are in this jam the best thing you can do is to acquaint yourself with the various methods that are advocated and, above all, to try to learn a bit more about yourself and how things work for you. The discussion of whether you are an A type or a B type of personality has far wider implications for your health than just the matter of smoking.

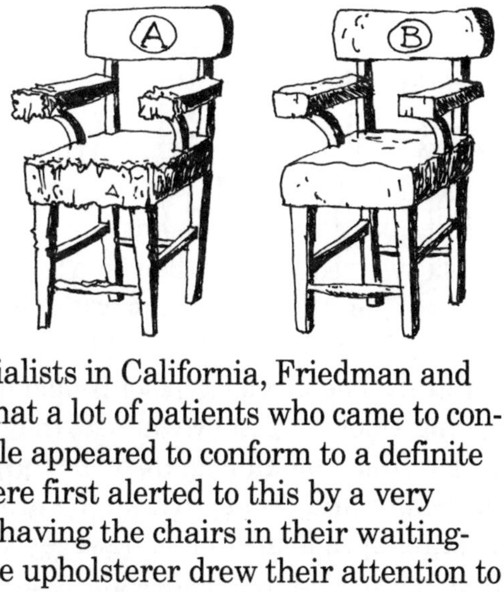

TYPES A AND B

In the 1950s two heart specialists in California, Friedman and Rosenman, became aware that a lot of patients who came to consult them about heart trouble appeared to conform to a definite type of personality. They were first alerted to this by a very strange incident: they were having the chairs in their waiting-room re-upholstered, and the upholsterer drew their attention to the fact that these chairs were worn only on the front edge. This implied that many of their patients were the type of people who could not sit comfortably and relaxed while waiting but were sitting on the edge of their chairs to get the appointment over and then to dash away. Interviews with their heart patients confirmed that they definitely belonged to the type of person who is impatient, hard driving, restless, aggressive and ambitious. They called this sort of person Type A.

Now it might conceivably have been that heart trouble rendered people impatient, hard driving, etc. rather than that this type of behaviour caused heart trouble, so Friedman and Rosenman had to study healthy people before any heart trouble had developed. In order to test this they assembled a group of 3,154 healthy men and assessed them as to whether they conformed to the A Type; these men were followed up for eight years, at the end of which it turned out that having A Type behaviour doubled a man's risk of having a first heart attack and more than doubled his risk of a second one.

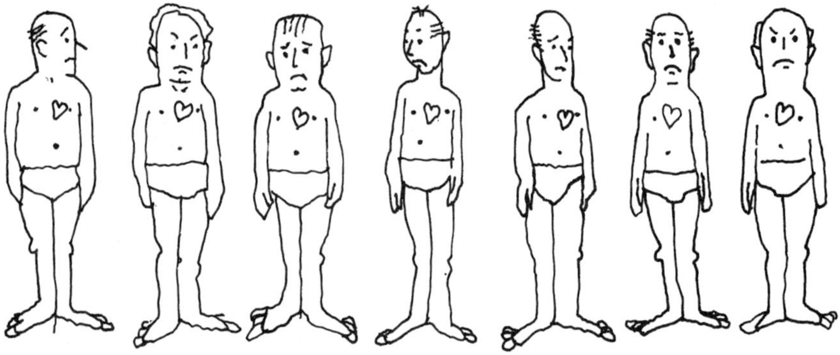

This study was carried out with men only because at that time men were much more prone to have heart attacks than women, but the same results also seemed to apply to women. It should be noted that nowadays the incidence of heart trouble in women is greater, and this may be the result of women increasingly coming out of the home and taking their place in the competitive, stressful world of men where A Type behaviour is common.

It should be noted that such research into the association between personality type and heart trouble in no way invalidates the work that has shown that a diet rich in cholesterol tends to produce heart attacks. But it seems clear that if A Type people and B Types (the B Type is the opposite of the A Type) are living on precisely the same diet, it is the former who will be more prone to heart attacks.

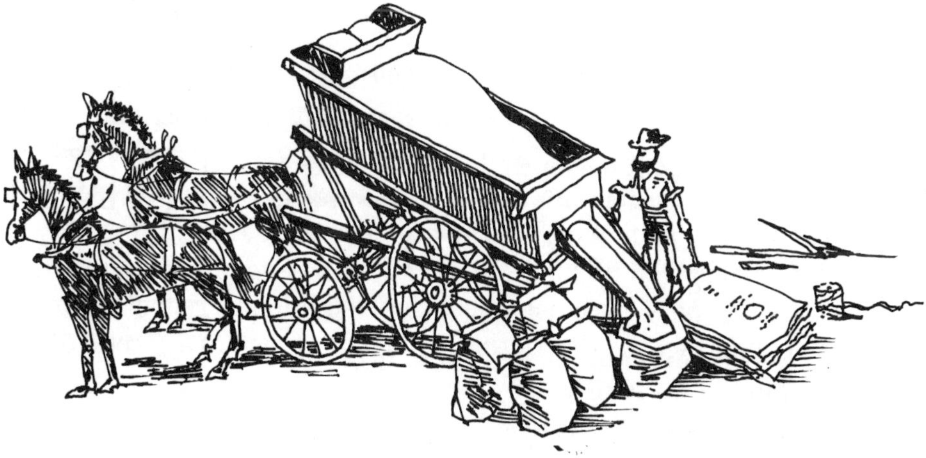

Friedman and Rosenman point out that heart trouble is very rare among the Amish communities. These are people in certain rural parts of America who eschew all the modern trappings of civilization – motor cars, electricity, television, etc. – and live very quiet, simple lives on their farms. Yet they live on a diet that has plenty of animal fat in it, as our farming ancestors did, and should therefore be specially liable to heart trouble.

As mentioned above, the B Type of behaviour is the opposite of the A Type: it implies patience, low competitiveness, retreat from confrontation, no outward expression of anger or hostility, and general denial of hassle or conflict, a somewhat 'Polyanna-ish' behaviour. If you are interested in how far you personally conform to the A Type or the B Type of personality you might like to try filling in the following questionnaire and seeing how you score.

QUESTIONNAIRE

Answer each question responding 'Yes' or 'No' by putting a tick in the appropriate column. In some cases you may have difficulty in deciding, but choose the alternative that is the more appropriate for most situations.

	YES	NO
1. Do you find it very irritating to have to wait in queues?	☐	☐
2. Do you find it too much trouble to make a fuss when you get really bad service in shops?	☐	☐
3. Are you quite proud of being a forceful, energetic person?	☐	☐
4. Do you think that there is little to complain of in the world today?	☐	☐
5. Does slackness in public servants impel you to make a protest?	☐	☐
6. Are you very seldom anxious, worried or upset?	☐	☐
7. Would you like to have litter-louts and vandals severely punished?	☐	☐
8. Were you rather too easy-going to be much of a success in your career?	☐	☐
9. Are you by nature rather rapid in your speech writing and movements?	☐	☐
10. On the whole, do you enjoy pretty good health and have few fears for the future?	☐	☐

The questionnaire is scored as follows: you add up all the 'Yes' answers given to the odd-numbered items, and the 'No' answers to the even-numbered, and thus the final score can be anything between 0 and 10. High scores indicate an A tendency and low scores a B tendency. Whatever score you have obtained don't take it too seriously for this questionnaire is given to you just to illustrate the sorts of behaviour and attitude that make up the two contrasting types of personality.

The heart specialists Friedman and Rosenman who originated this concept reasoned that if they could give therapy to people with an extreme A Type response they could get them to modify their habitual behaviour and thus be less liable to have a heart attack, or if they had already had one attack it would lower the risk of their having another. They have published material showing that they have had some success in their therapeutic efforts. These doctors rather idealized the B Type of personality and implied that we should all aim to live our lives as much in accordance with this ideal as we can. Alas, other researchers were later to show that the extreme B Type were specially prone to another sort of disease – cancer!

It has long been known that people of a certain type of personality are specially prone to develop cancer, but what this personality characteristic is has always been rather vague. Some doctors have spoken of cancer patients as being rather 'nice' people. The research that gave more definite information began with the investigation of personality using a questionnaire, the *Eysenck Personality Inventory*, that gives a score on 'neuroticism' as well as other scales. If someone gets a high 'neuroticism' score it does not mean that they are in any way mentally ill, but that they have a tendency to be over-emotional and 'highly strung'. Such a score is obtained by the person admitting to items like 'Does your mood often go up and down?', 'Would you call yourself a nervous person?', 'Do you worry a lot about your looks?', 'Have you ever wished that you were dead?' This questionnaire has been given to thousands of people in all walks of life, and ordinary normal people can be expected to get a modest score on the neuroticism scale, and those who are very 'highly strung' rather a high score – as do patients in a state of anxiety.

This questionnaire was given to a group of patients before any diagnosis was made about their condition and the surprising fact emerged that many of those who had an abnormally low score on the 'neuroticism' scale were later found to be suffering from cancer. The research was extended and it was repeatedly found that cancer victims tended to have a remarkably low 'neuroticism' score. An abnormally low score results from their denying just about every item that referred to them having any troubles in life. Their responses were just too good to be true! They have been described as being: 'over-cooperative, appeasing, unassertive, over-patient, avoiding conflict, seeking harmony, compliant, with a defensive response to stress, and a failure to express negative emotions like anger and anxiety openly.' They are, in fact, very like the B Type that Friedman and Rosenman idealized because it was not associated with heart disease.

Further work by a number of different doctors and psychologists showed that the original conception of the A Type personality in relation to vulnerability to heart disease was rather flawed. It was not so much the tendency to be hurried, impatient and ambitious that led to trouble with the heart and arteries, but the anger that is engendered in some (but not all) people by frustration of go-getting behaviour. Anger produces excess quantities of certain hormones being discharged into the blood, and this may result in processes that lead to blood-clots and the narrowing of the arteries. A doctor in Yugoslavia, Ronald Grossarth-Maticek, developed his own measures of personality based on previous work by other people, and produced some truly remarkable data showing the connection between personality measures of what he called 'cancer proneness' and the patients' subsequent death by cancer. Similarly, his personality measures of proneness to Coronary Heart Disease (CHD) and stroke also predicted death from these disorders. A very simplified summary of some of his results is shown in the figure below.

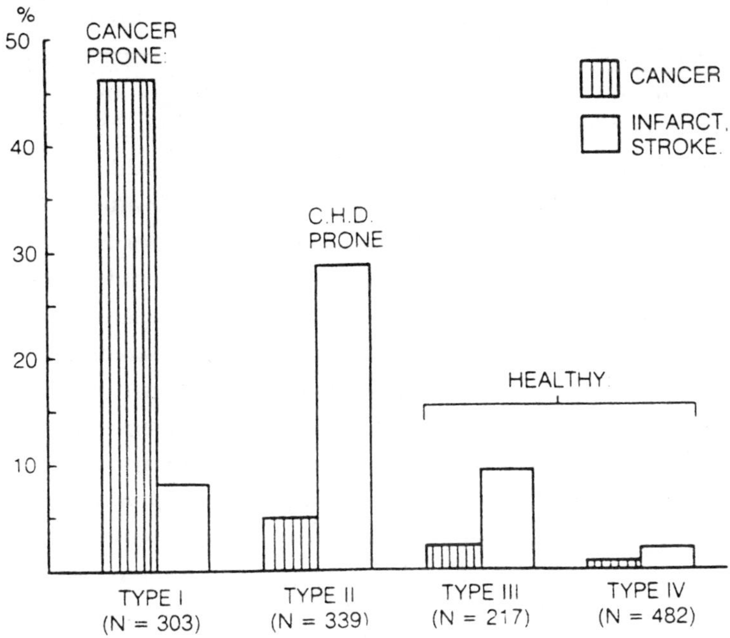

FIG. 5.1 *Deaths from cancer and CHD according to personality type; Yugoslav study*

Reproduced from *Rebel with a Cause: The Autobiography of Hans Eysenck* by kind permission of the author.

What was done in this Yugoslav study was to assemble an experimental population of 1,341 people who had no pathological symptoms at the time and classify them into four groups on the basis of the personality measures that emerged from psychological testing. Type I were diagnosed as being cancer-prone, Type II as being CHD prone, and Types III and IV were of normal personality (i.e. between the extremes of I and II) but Type III were rather odd sort of people and it was suspected that they might develop disease. After 10 years had passed these individuals were located, and as you can see from the figure, 50% of the cancer-prone people had died of cancer, and nearly 30% of the CHD prone people had died of the relevant disease, in contrast to the small percentage of each type who had died of the non-relevant disease. The personality oddity of Type III was slightly related to a higher death-rate than that of the normal people of Type IV.

These figures seem almost too good to be true, and indeed the whole research of Grossarth-Maticek has come under considerable criticism, especially from doctors in Germany. One of the puzzles is that although it is perfectly reasonable to expect people of Type A personality (his Type II) to be specially liable to heart attacks, there is no sort of rationale linking the contrary type with proneness to cancer. For Type A people their habitual impatience and anger at frustration certainly produce hormonal changes in the bloodstream, and hence clotting and obstruction of arteries; in addition, they tend to go on exerting themselves when they are completely exhausted and should rest, thus placing an intolerable strain on the heart. But as yet we do not know what causes cancer to develop (except in response to local irritation and trauma) and there seems to be absolutely no rationale for linking susceptibility to this disease to one type of personality. The statistical link with Type B personality that has sometimes been observed is a complete mystery, and some people hold that it is a fluke.

I do not propose to go into all the details of the controversy that has arisen around this work; it is presented here as an example of the sort of research that has developed out of the original work in the 1950s on the A Type and B Type of personality in California. Grossarth-Maticek went on to investigate how best to proceed with cancer-prone and CHD-prone patients so that their tendency was minimized and they did not eventually develop the disease in a fatal form. This involved trying to get them to modify their habitual life-style in ways that were indicated by previous research.

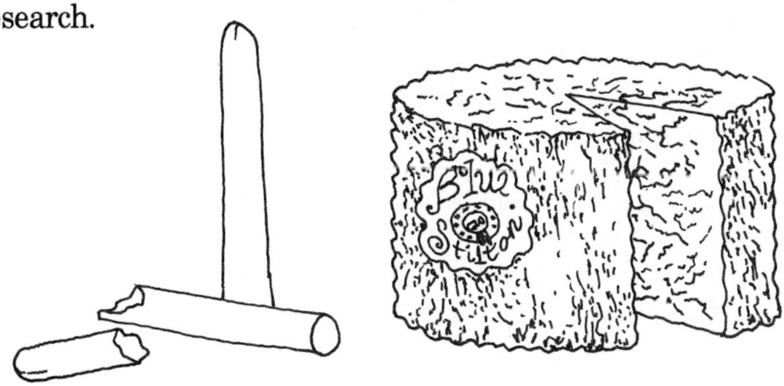

THE IMPLICATIONS OF PERSONALITY TYPE

This is a book about health and not about disease, and is addressed to the majority of people in later life who are moderately fit and aim to remain so. You may therefore wonder why I have digressed above and discussed the extremes of ill-health and the personality attributes of those who suffer from it – most of them in the researches discussed were not old at all. I have made this digression for several reasons.

It is important to realize that people are very different, and it is unwise to generalize too much about prescriptions for health. A lifestyle that suits one type of person may not suit another. While some people would be better if they slowed themselves down, others should consider how they might pep themselves up and face life's challenges in a more active way. In the years after retirement people have less need to be ambitious, hard-driving and competitive, and if they know that they suffer from heart trouble they should study how to arrange their lives in a more leisurely manner.

Similarly the opposite type should remember that it is not healthy to coddle yourself too much. As pointed out in another chapter of this book an adequate amount of exercise is essential for us all in later life, and research studies have shown that perhaps the majority of older people do not take enough. The medical advice that used to be given to people with heart conditions is now acknowledged to have been wrong; even if you have a dickey heart, it does it good to make it race a little within moderation. It will soon tell you when to stop and rest.

Physical exercise apart, you should not consider that now you have reached a certain age you should retire into your chimney corner and hide from the challenges of life or murmur that, 'You can't teach an old dog new tricks'; as one experienced psychologist has put it 'When the mind ceases to deal with novelty the body begins to die.'

In another book of mine about older people* I have referred to them as being variously 'Task-oriented' or 'Lotos-eaters', these two types being rather vaguely related to the A Type and B Type of personality. Provided that you do not veer too far to the extreme of either you should stay healthy. All the work that has been done on personality type implies that to some extent at least it is genetically determined, and that you are stuck with the basic type your parents gave you, but no-one challenges the fact that environmental influences are very powerful in modifying your habitual behaviour. We all like to say with Popeye 'I yam what I yam!' but all the work that has been discussed above has shown that a deliberate programme of behaviour modification can definitely affect people's life-styles to the betterment of their health. You should be the expert on you, and with knowledge understand how best to steer a course of life between the rocks.

---

* *On the Tip of Your Tongue; Your Memory in Later Life* by H B Gibson. Third Age Press. 1995.

DISABILITY IN LATER LIFE

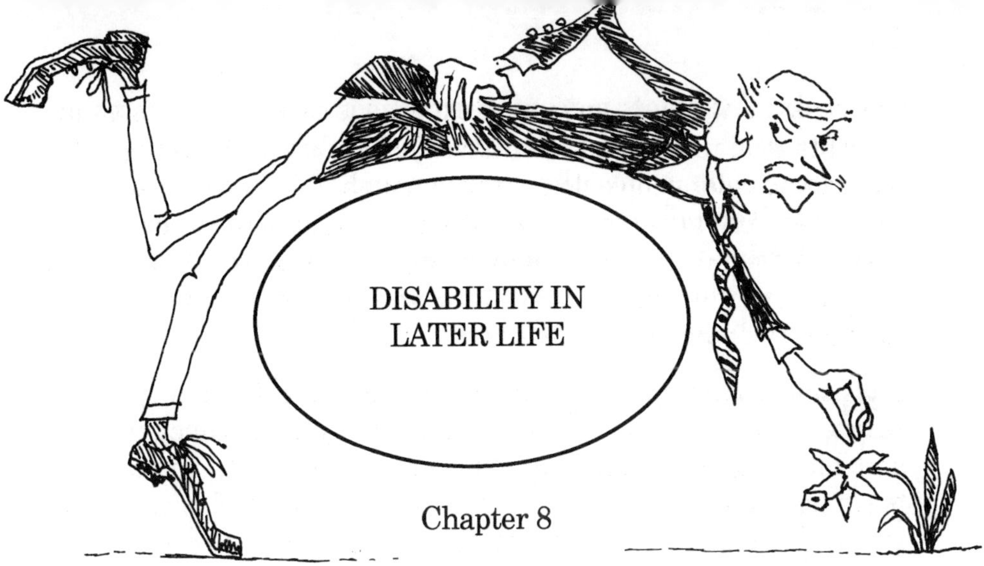

Chapter 8

While you may be pretty fit and retain your health by sensible living, no-one is immune from the effects of various mistakes that were made in designing the human frame when Adam was on the drawing-board, many of which were passed on to Eve via his rib, with a few added. You may develop some disability such as an arthritic hip or a dickey heart while you remain otherwise in pretty good health. This chapter is about the more common of these conditions and what you can do to prevent or mitigate their results.

It has long been observed that if lay people read about a variety of diseases and disorders, say, in a medical text-book, they then begin to imagine that they are suffering from all sorts of things and feel distinctly unwell; you should not assume it's inevitable you'll develop any condition described in this book which is, after all, about health and staying well.

FRACTURES AND OSTEOPOROSIS

The incidence of fractures of the thigh-bone due to falls is small and preventable – up to 2% in men and 3% in women before the age of 75. The higher percentage in women is due to the fact that they are more prone to develop osteoporosis after the menopause. However, you may have this condition and never have such an accident if you take proper care. Such factors as proper footwear, a stair-case that is properly lighted and free from hazards, noting when the pavements are icy and slippery, avoiding carrying bulky loads when bicycling, are all matters of importance in preventing falls. New evidence shows that practising T'ai Chi or some other form of balance training may also be effective. It may be noted that up to the age of about 55 men are more prone to incur fractures than women, because they tend to lead more dangerous lives than women, both at work and in their leisure. The effects of breaking a thigh-bone on frail older people can be very serious indeed, and it is worth-while considering if you are at risk.

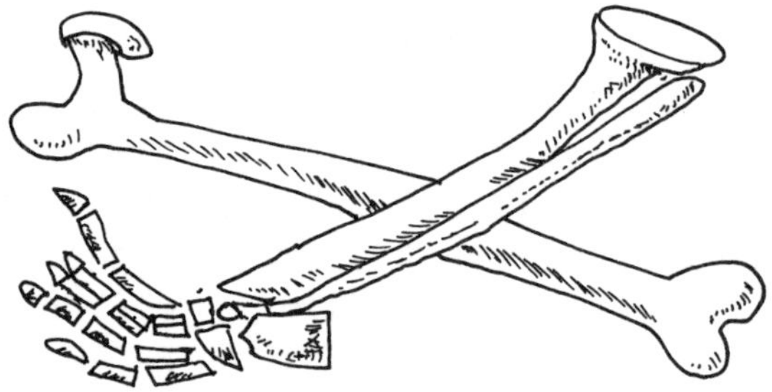

Osteoporosis is due to a very strange feature of the human skeleton. The hard tissue of bones is constantly being re-absorbed and replaced, and osteoporosis occurs when the replacement process does not keep pace with the re-absorption. The bones become brittle and snap easily under violent stress. It is not known just how the hormones affect this process, but women are prone to develop the disorder with the alteration of the hormone balance after the menopause and if they have had their ovaries surgically removed. Hormone replacement therapy, which is now widely practised but is a matter for strict medical control, has been found to decrease the incidence of fractures.

The thigh-bone is not the only part of the skeleton that is affected by osteoporosis of course, the bones of the fore-arm and the spinal vertebrae are also notably affected. The condition of 'dowager's hump' is mainly due to degeneration of the spine and rib-cage, although why it is attributed particularly to dowagers is a mystery.

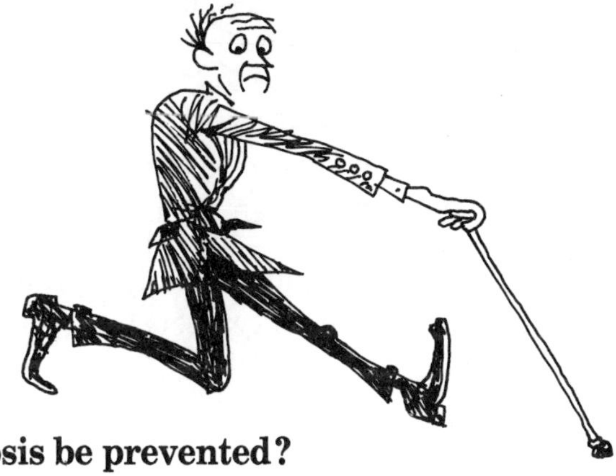

Can osteoporosis be prevented?

The answer must be 'no' and 'yes'. The chief factors that you can't do anything about are as follows: being of European or Asiatic race; having a slender body-build; being a woman; having had ovaries removed; being elderly. The main things you can do something about are: having a sensible mixed diet; avoiding drinking too much alcohol; avoiding smoking; taking an adequate amount of exercise. Unfortunately most of the precautions that can be taken refer very much to the younger years of life when a sturdy skeleton should be built up; however, it is never too late to check at least some of the ravages of an unwise life-style and it has been shown that an improvement in fitness can be achieved into the 80s or even 90s through regular exercise, such as walking. As for hormone replacement therapy, that is a matter you must discuss with your doctor.

Here is some good news for those who consider that they have a 'weight problem'. Those who are comfortably plump are less at risk from fractures due to falls than those who are elegantly thin. Not only are those of a substantial body-build less subject to osteoporosis, but if the body is properly cushioned with fat the bones are less likely to break in a fall. While fatness to the degree of obesity is certainly to be avoided on general health grounds, there are some benefits to be derived from being chubby.

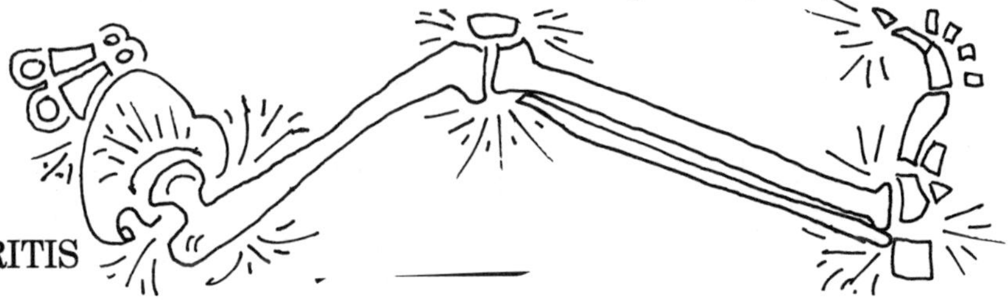

ARTHRITIS

Arthritis refers to abnormal and generally painful conditions of the joints, and there are three main types: osteoarthritis, rheumatoid arthritis and gout.

Osteoarthritis

This condition may affect all the joints of the body but it is especially serious for the load-bearing joints, the hips and the knees. The disorder is due to the partial destruction of the layer of cartilage that covers the ends of the bones and ensures a smooth movement of the joint, and it is not at all clear why it comes about.

Obviously the amount of weight borne by the joint has something to do with its degeneration, for obese people are particularly subject to it, but there may be some additional factor that causes both obesity and the degeneration of the joints. Where it is the knee joints that are affected there is some evidence that it is more prevalent in those who have had heavy jobs involving much knee-bending. It is a disease of later life, of course, because like any other machine the body is subject to wear and tear, and these weight-bearing joints have had a hard time, although most of us manage to maintain adequate repair.

About 5% of people over the age of 55 will have trouble due to osteoarthritis in the knees, and a slightly smaller proportion in the hips. The disease generally makes its presence known by pain on movement, and it may also be detected by x-raying the joint. Curiously, there is not a close correspondence between the amount of pain felt and the amount of damage that is evident on x-ray examination. Thus in one study in the 75+ group of men 20.5% showed some signs of the disease in the knees but only 4.5% complained of it; the figures for women were respectively 41.8% and 13.8%. Where knees are concerned women are rather more affected than men in later life, but it is not clear whether this has anything to do with the changes in hormone balance after the menopause. As far as I know no-one has published research on osteoarthritis relating to hormone replacement therapy.

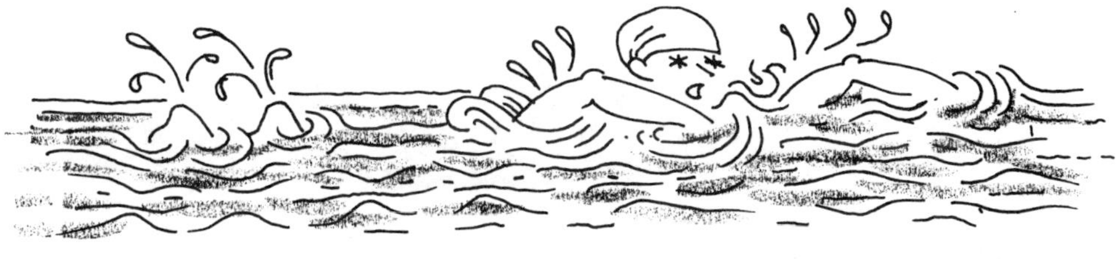

As to prevention it is largely a matter of looking back in sorrow. People need to avoid obesity in their younger years and also refrain from putting excessive strain on their joints. In later life people still need to avoid obesity, and if they become aware of an osteoarthritic condition to avoid carrying weights. Swimming becomes the exercise of choice because the body is supported in water.

The replacement of knees and hips by artificial joints has now become a common and very successful operation. The techniques involved are continually developing and we may expect further improvements.

Rheumatoid arthritis

This form of arthritis can effect any joint but mainly attacks the arms and hands. It is not due to a breakdown of the cartilage but a pathological growth of the membrane lining the joint. It is not specially a disease of later life and some people may have a life-long battle with it. About the most that can be done for it is to suppress pain by analgesics and attempt to preserve function by physiotherapy. There are treatments involving steroids, gold injections and drugs, but the benefits that are to be derived from these must be balanced against the unpleasant side-effects. Surgical treatment may sometimes be necessary.

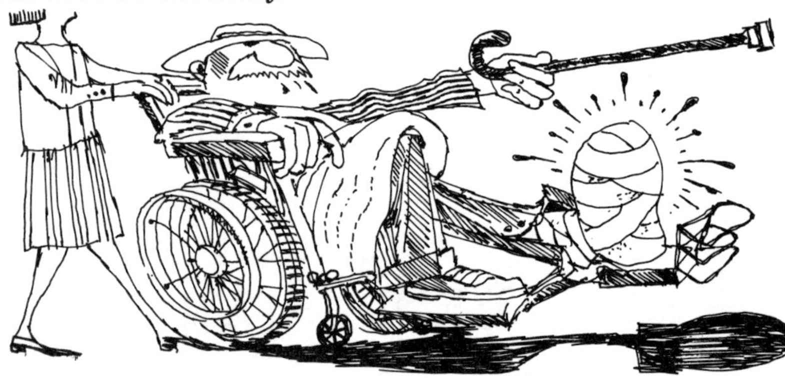

Gout

This is caused by a build-up of tiny crystals of uric acid in the joints, and usually affects the feet and hands. The whole flesh around the joint may become hot, inflamed and sore. Some individuals have a propensity to develop gout in later life and it may be triggered by eating certain foods that are rich in purine, a chemical that gives rise to excessive uric acid. These foods are notably oily fish, liver and kidneys, and beans. If you have experienced the condition you will learn just what foods you personally should avoid. As well as certain foods heavy red wines such as port may bring on gout, and have given rise to the stereotype of the rich elderly gentleman with his bandaged gouty foot resting on a footstool. The condition is normally self-limiting and lasts only a few days at a time.

CHRONIC BRONCHITIS

Chronic bronchitis can be a serious problem in later life and comes high on the list of the killing diseases. On common-sense grounds we might expect the incidence of this disorder to have steadily increased over the last few decades as the Jeremiahs keep telling us how the planet Earth is getting steadily more polluted so that soon we won't have enough breathable air around.

However the statistics about death from bronchitis are surprising: in 1963 the total deaths from the disease were 30,001 in England and Wales, but this rate of mortality has steadily declined so that in 1990 there were only 4,934. Some interesting facts emerge which may help you to plan the best ways of avoiding this dangerous condition.

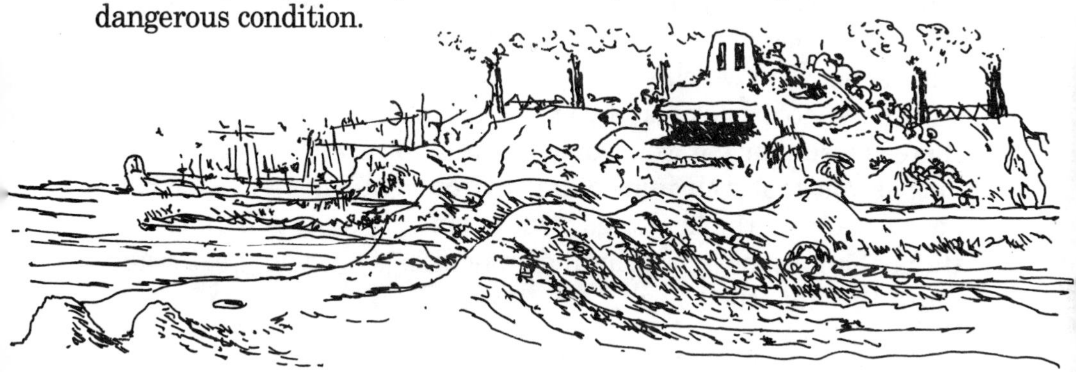

Chronic bronchitis, like many other diseases that may attack us in the Third Age, is associated with some factors that we can't do much about, and some that we can. We need to face the latter part of our lives with strong and healthy lungs, but if in childhood bad living conditions and poor diet produced many chest infections, the adults who had grown up with weak chests would be subject later on to chronic bronchitis.

Thus, those who were born at the beginning of this century would more often have unhealthy childhoods, so by the time they reached the age of retirement around 1963 would be very vulnerable to bronchitis and likely to be included in the 30,001 deaths from that disease for that year. The continuous fall in the mortality rates for bronchitis has thus reflected the steady increase of childhood health during the century. A second reason that accounts for the decreased bronchitis in men is the fall in cigarette smoking in the second half of this century; unfortunately, women have not reduced their smoking proportionately.

You can't do anything about your childhood health now, and you really can't do much about the air-pollution that surrounds you, except by joining a clean-air pressure group or packing up your home and moving to a rural environment where the atmosphere is purer. Surprisingly, although atmospheric pollution is a cause of bronchitis, it is not a particularly strong factor in adult life. If you live in a village in a part of the country where the air is very pure but the house in which you live has someone who fills the air with a fug of tobacco smoke, and you spend time in a club or pub where there is a similar fug, you would be better off living in a city as long as you kept your immediate environment smoke-free. When people consider the health hazards of smoking they generally think of lung cancer, but chronic bronchitis is an even greater and direct threat to their health.

One way of lowering the risk of developing bronchitis is to ask your doctor for an immunization injection against 'flu. Every year there is a minor epidemic of 'flu in the winter months and some doctors advise that everyone over the age of 65 should have such an immunization annually in the early autumn. All measures should be taken to avoid getting run down by colds; do not try to economize on heating – never let yourself get too cold. One of the disadvantages of ageing for many people is that they fail to detect a lowering of their body-temperature as they did when younger. You should live in a warm, dry place, and you should not put up with living quarters that are cold and damp, for you have as much right to live in a healthy environment as has your local housing officer.

Make a fuss if your home is sub-standard in respect of this essential matter; perhaps some part of the annual toll of deaths every winter is due to the long-suffering humility of too many pensioners.

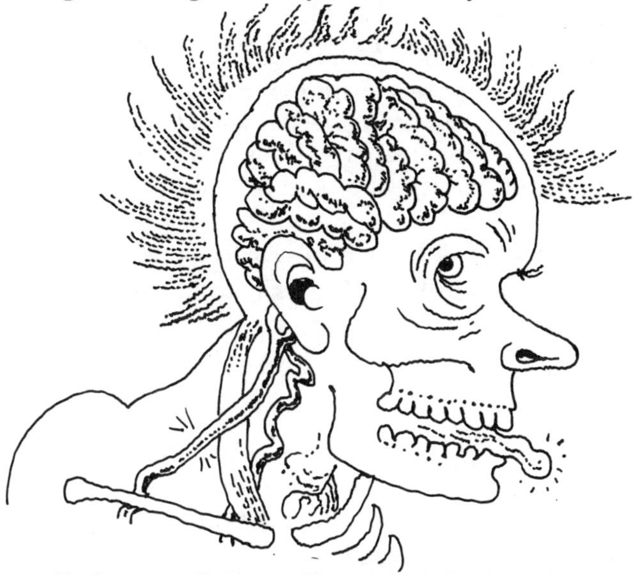

STROKE

The term stroke is applied to conditions of loss of brain function that are due to something interfering with the brain's normal blood-supply of more than transitory duration. A stroke may be caused by the breaking of blood vessels leading to bleeding either within the brain, or below the outer sheath that encloses the brain (the arachnoid membrane). In the latter case a large blood-clot forms that causes damaging pressure. Alternatively, some obstruction may cause a portion of the brain to be starved of blood (infarction) so it will cease to function and then die. There is also a condition that is transitory and lasts less than 24 hours, which is usually due to a small blood-clot, which obstructs the free flow of blood to the brain and thus interrupts the function of part of it for a while, causing temporary memory loss. This latter type of accident is familiarly known as TIA (transient ischaemic attack). If this occurs it should immediately be reported to the doctor who may initiate action designed to prevent further trouble. About

15 - 20% of strokes are heralded by TIA.

The above are broad general descriptions of what is meant by stroke, but there are many sub-divisions, and one medical writer, faced with the complexity of the many definitions, wrote:

> After all, these terms simply tell us how badly off the patient is; they say nothing about the mechanism of stroke. None of these categories approaches homogeneity; they contain fruits as divergent as grapes and watermelons.

The purpose of this chapter is to suggest how you may avoid the possible disabilities of later life, and what to do if they threaten, and so it is useful to have some understanding of how they come about. The incidence of stroke increases steadily as ageing advances, and once the conditions that produce it have set in there is no way (to date) of removing them from within the brain, as a plumber might clean out and replace defective pipes in a heating system, but you can take action to minimize the risk of these conditions developing.

The prevention of high blood-pressure (hypertension) is one of the obvious measures to take, too much pressure in the blood-vessels may rupture their walls. It has been found that middle-aged people suffering from serious hypertension are three times as likely to have a stroke in the next 24 years as those with normal blood-pressure.

However, even a moderate degree of hypertension is a risk factor in middle-age, and it is never too late to take active steps to reduce the pressure. Drug treatment of those at risk under the age of 65 significantly reduces the incidence of stroke occurring later on, but there are also many measures that may be taken independent of drugs.

The following risk factors and the ways to minimize them should be considered:

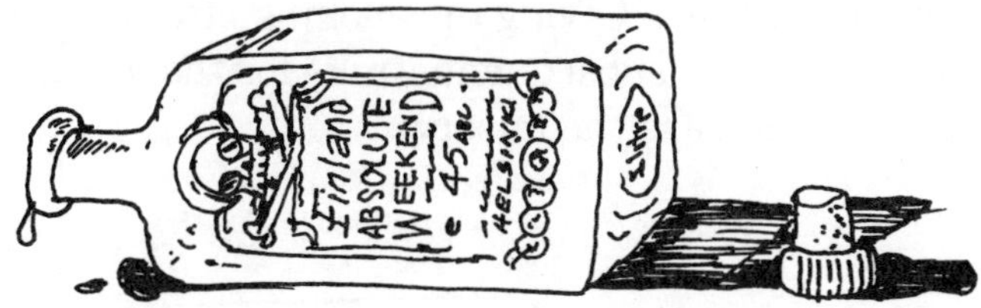

1. Alcohol

A high level of alcohol intake is a risk factor for stroke, but even moderate drinkers should be aware that a single incident of binge-drinking can send the blood-pressure through the roof and produce a stroke. This factor was discovered in Finland where it is the custom of men to go on the binge on Fridays and Saturdays, and hence produce a crop of strokes at the end of the week. However, it is not well validated for older people, possibly because senior citizens are less prone to indulge in orgies of drinking when out on the town. However, it is better to be safe than sorry, and it would be a shame to celebrate your sixty-fifth birthday by binge-drinking ('Just this once!') and be carried off to hospital on a stretcher.

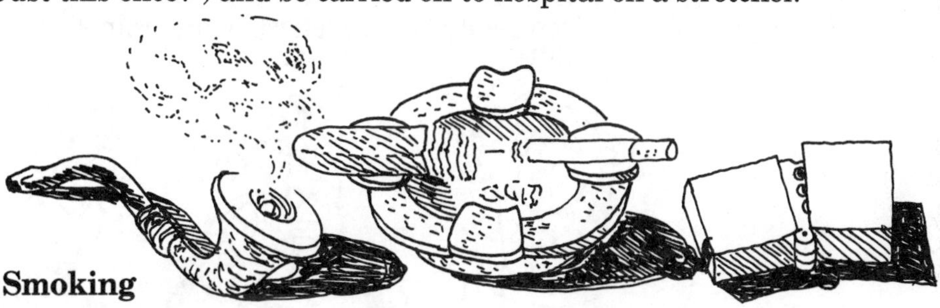

2. Smoking

Throughout this book you will have become accustomed to reading that smoking is one of the main villains of the piece in relation to various disabilities, and as the medical profession has been carrying on a crusade against it for some years you may expect to have it indicted in respect to stroke. As a matter of fact although smokers are rather more prone to suffer stroke than non-smokers, it is not a very strong risk-factor for those over the age of 65. Should those who have suffered a small stroke give up smoking? One eminent authority on the subject is quite indulgent with his patients and advises, 'Giving up smoking after a stroke is unlikely to reduce the risk of subsequent stroke for the average patient, and may just increase the misery.'

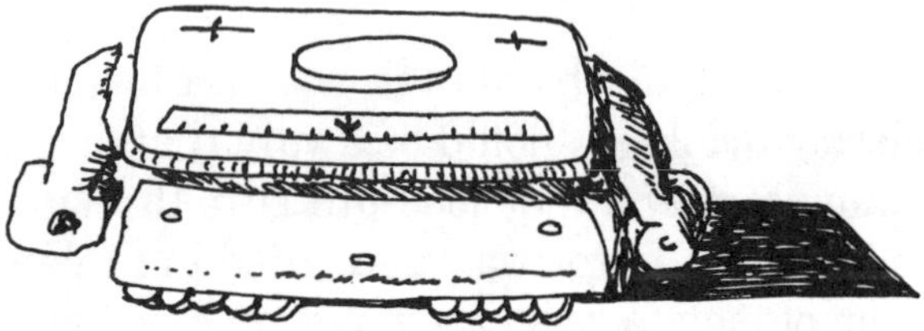

3. Obesity

Again, you may expect obesity to be heavily indicted in respect to stroke since it appears to be a causal factor in so many other disabilities of later life, but although there is a slightly greater risk of obese individuals incurring a stroke, there is little direct connection. Obesity may be responsible for both raising the blood-pressure and deterring people from taking enough physical exercise, and that indeed relates to proneness to die from stroke.

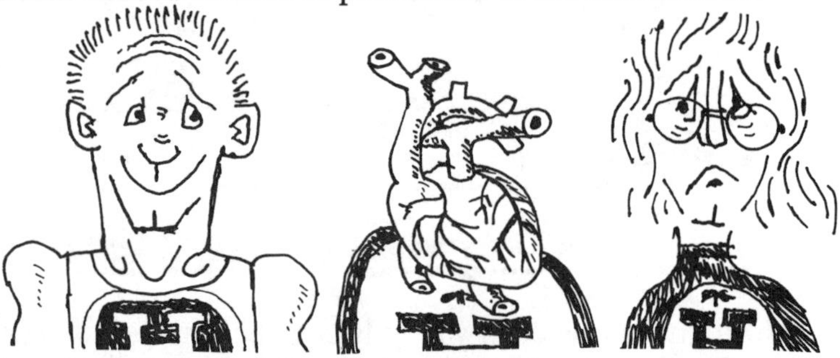

4. Exercise

Here the picture is not at all clear. It was found in a survey of 50,000 Harvard alumni that those who had participated in sports while at college had half the rate of fatal strokes in later years, compared with those who had not engaged in sports. Other studies have shown that a low degree of activity during leisure time does not increase the risk of suffering from stroke, but it increases the likelihood of dying from such an attack. It seems likely that those who sustain a stroke but recover from it are people in otherwise good health, taking an adequate amount of exercise is essential for retaining health in later life.

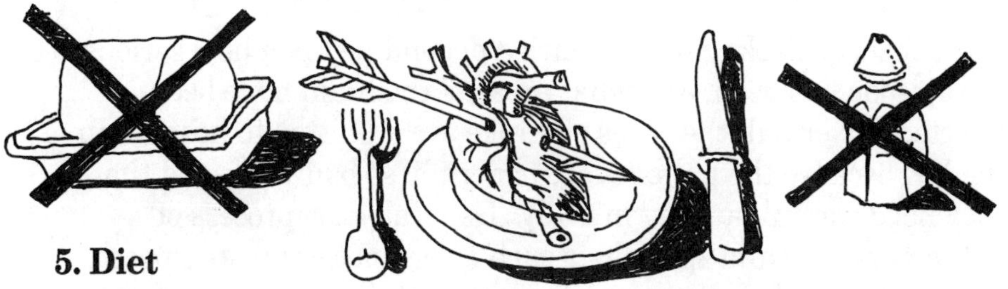

5. Diet

There are two risk factors in diet relating to proneness to stroke: foods containing a high amount of unsaturated fat, and common salt. The unsaturated fat gives rise to a sort of 'gunge' (atheroma) that may be deposited on the walls of the arteries, and pieces may flake off to cause an obstruction and hence infarction in the brain as described earlier. This type of stroke and coronary heart disease are related in that they are both due to atheroma in the arteries. Salt has the property of raising the blood-pressure and it should therefore be used sparingly in cooking and not be sprinkled lavishly on food at the dinner table.

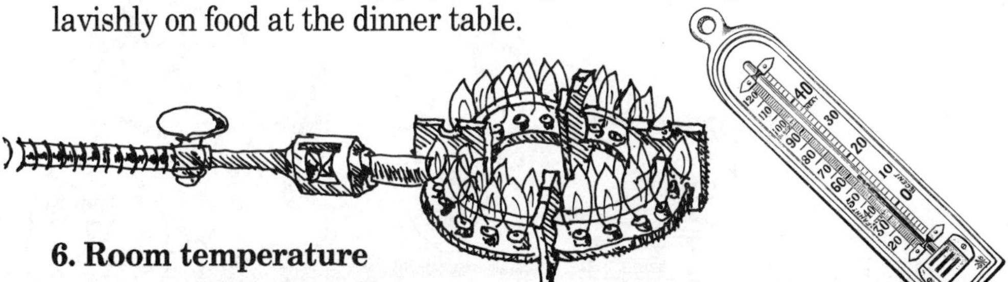

6. Room temperature

There appears to be a relationship between extremes of temperature and risk of stroke; swings between being very hot and very cold produce swings in blood-pressure, and thus may precipitate stroke. As pointed out earlier, in later life there is a reduced perception of temperature and so homes should be kept evenly warm all the time.

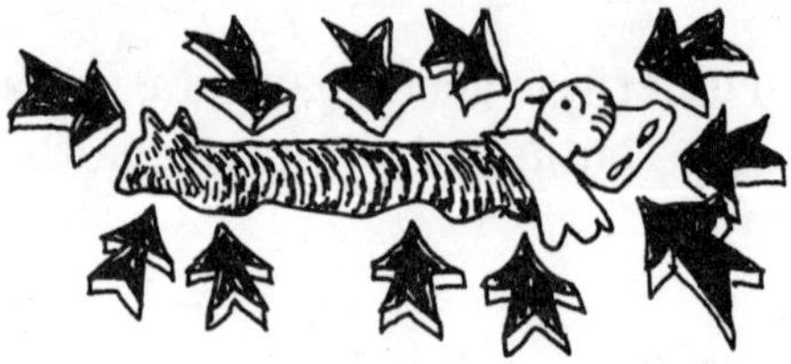

Therapy after a stroke

The effects of stroke are very varied depending upon how serious the episode has been, and what areas of the brain have been affected. Over half the cases of stroke are admitted to hospital in the UK because the patients are generally so badly affected that they need careful nursing initially. Generally the process of recovery is slow and specialists such as physiotherapists, speech therapists, psychologists, and occupational therapists may be involved in the rehabilitation of the patient. What is needed for recovery above all things is a strong determination on the part of the patient to regain as much as possible of his or her normal functions, and their family should be actively involved in all rehabilitative measures.

A final note: recent research has shown the benefits of taking a small (150 mg) dose of aspirin daily to prevent the blood becoming too viscous.

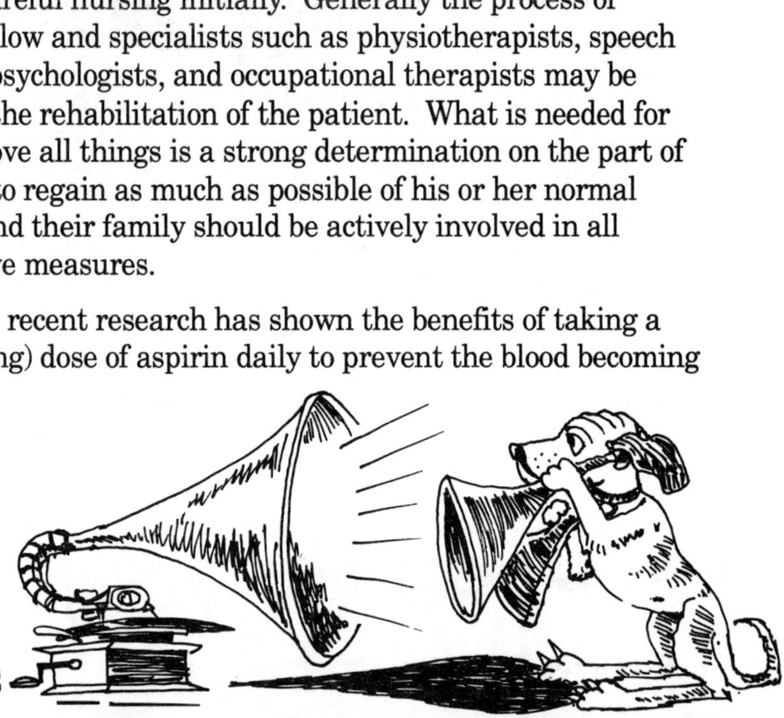

DEAFNESS

Deafness is a 'hidden handicap': it may not be obvious at first that someone is not hearing properly and so it may appear that they are stupid, and it is sometimes the cause of people becoming socially isolated. Traditionally it has become part of the stereotype of a foolish old person: Eric Midwinter refers ironically to 'the doddering loon, slumped with listless ear-trumpet, over the board table', in his depiction of this popular image of an elderly member of a council. It is no wonder therefore, that some people try to conceal their deafness.

Alex Comfort, writing in 1990, reckoned that out of 1,300,000 deaf people over the age of 65 in Britain, only 400,000 had hearing aids. It is hoped that the position is improving as people now entering the Third Age are showing more determination to combat the negative consequences of ageism.

The various reasons for the decline in hearing in later life are very complex and are described by Lorraine Jeffrey in her book listed in Appendix B. Free hearing-aids are available on the National Health after testing when patients have been referred to audiology clinics by their GPs. Because of financial constraints, the NHS hearing-aids are pretty basic: they magnify sound and in some circumstances make strong background noises too loud causing speech to be distorted and difficult to understand. If you wish to obtain a more sophisticated type of instrument which will be adapted to fit your particular type of hearing problem, it would be unwise just to buy one of the many models that are advertised in magazines and elsewhere. You should consult your local audiology clinic who will give you independent advice as to where to go for further professional help. It is strange that nowadays everyone accepts that their vision may be constantly changing with age and so they go to the optician for periodic check-ups, but they have yet to realize that much the same thing happens to their hearing.

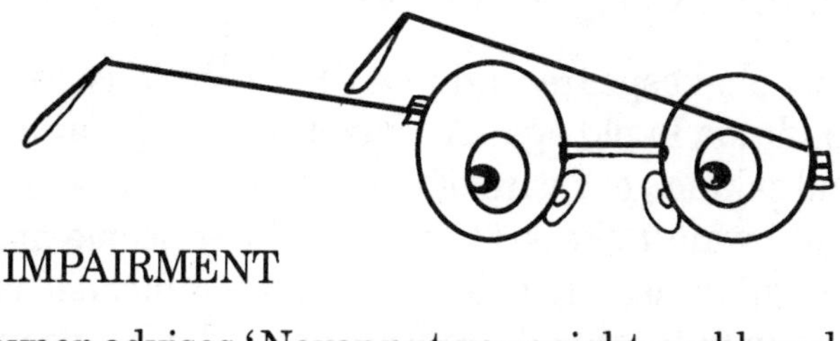

VISUAL IMPAIRMENT

Claire Rayner advises 'Never put your sight problem down to "old age" and ignore it.' While most people will experience some deterioration in their sight in old age, there is a difference between this, which can be corrected with spectacles, and an eye disease which may need other treatment. The most common conditions in later life are:

Cataracts – a cloudy film obscures vision. Over 120,000 people, most of them elderly, are successfully operated on every year to replace the faulty lens with a man-made substitute.

Macular degeneration – central vision is gradually lost, in one eye at a time, but sufferers of this condition seldom go completely blind. Most can learn to use the remaining peripheral vision to get around and aids, such as magnifiers, are also a help.

Glaucoma – is the result of excess pressure from the watery fluid in the eye which is normally drained away. If not treated, it will damage your vision. Regular eye tests are essential, especially if you have a relative with the condition, but if you have sudden changes in your vision, such as seeing coloured halos around lights, you should seek immediate help. Glaucoma is treatable with eye-drops, tablets or surgery.

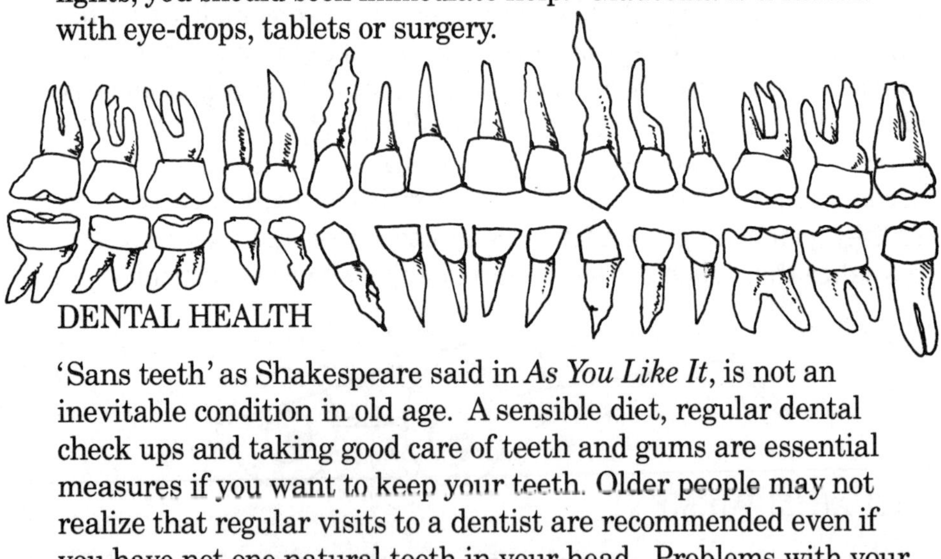

DENTAL HEALTH

'Sans teeth' as Shakespeare said in *As You Like It*, is not an inevitable condition in old age. A sensible diet, regular dental check ups and taking good care of teeth and gums are essential measures if you want to keep your teeth. Older people may not realize that regular visits to a dentist are recommended even if you have not one natural tooth in your head. Problems with your gums and persistent mouth ulcers should always be treated before they lead to something more serious. Fluoridation in water supplies and improved diets for most children mean that many youngsters are cavity-free. The dental problems of most older people are probably legacies of their childhood but cutting down on sweet foods and fizzy drinks and the use of a toothpaste with fluoride will help preserve what's left.

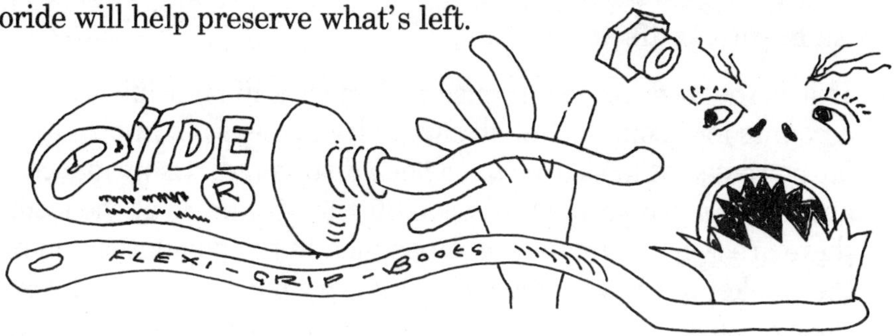

DEMENTIA AND PSEUDO-DEMENTIA

Like stroke, dementia is due to physical injury to the brain due to violence or disease, and it can occur at any age due to an accident (such as a car crash), poisoning, infection, or bio-chemical disorder, but it is much more common in later life. Dementia may be defined as a general impairment of the function of the brain in thinking, learning and remembering, and in its extreme forms sufferers are rendered incapable of looking after themselves. There are two main types: vascular dementia, which is closely allied to stroke, and Alzheimer's disease.

Vascular dementia

This is due to repeated small breaks in the blood-vessels of the brain due to some of the reasons that produce a stroke, and although some individuals have a natural vulnerability it is partly preventable by attending to the measures to prevent stroke as described earlier. The condition can sometimes be halted for a while by remedial therapy, such as keeping the blood-pressure down, but this form of dementia often leads to an early death.

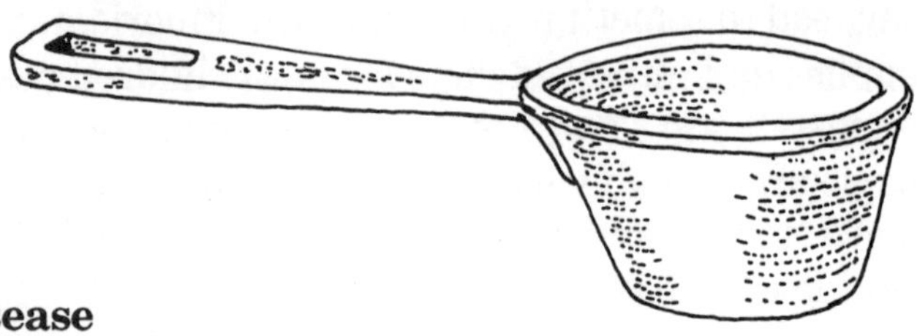

Alzheimer's disease

This is the most common cause of dementia in later life and accounts for about 70% of all cases. Its cause is not known and so far no remedial measures have been discovered. Its incidence is about 2% in people aged between 65 and 75, and as at the latter age there are twice as many women as men in the population (many of the weaker sex having died off) it is very much a female disease in the older age group. In the very old group – those over 85 – the incidence is about 20%.

As little can be done about it in the present state of medical science, we might say, 'Why worry? We have got to die of something'. However, sufferers can live for quite a few years with the brain steadily deteriorating, and they pose a problem for their carers. The disease is a cause for concern for many people who haven't got it and never will have, but when they find themselves getting a bit forgetful they fear that they are in the first stages of the disease.

Because of this widespread worry it is indeed a problem for the community, and Lord Butterfield has gone on record as saying that investigation of dementia should be a major objective for medicine for the coming century. The medical and allied professions have indeed embarked on a considerable research programme concerned with Alzheimer's disease in the UK. There are currently 30 research projects, which have discovered some very useful facts: it used to be thought that eating food prepared in aluminium vessels put one at risk for developing it, but later research has failed to show that there is a definite association. Some, but not all cases have been shown to have a genetic link, and there is evidence that it may be connected genetically with Down's syndrome. The genetic predisposition to develop the disease is certainly not strong, and no one should be concerned if they have a relative who is afflicted.

Because there are many conditions, both organic and functional, that mimic the first stages of the disease, diagnosis is not easy and can only be achieved by exclusion. Many people are confused as to what Alzheimer's disease means: it refers to a condition in which there have been certain structural changes in the brain tissue, and unless such changes have occurred the patient has not got AD whatever else may be wrong. Until comparatively recent years there used to be some confusion over the diagnosis of Alzheimer's disease, and there was a risk of false diagnosis, but early in the 1990s guidelines were developed. It is now held that we should consider three categories, definite, probable and possible. A definite diagnosis is only possible when actual evidence of structural change has been obtained as well as all the indicative data about the patient's behaviour and capabilities. Proof of such anatomical changes can only be obtained normally by examining the brain post mortem, but it is possible to do a biopsy – that is, obtaining a tiny sample of the brain by a penetrative technique. Biopsies are seldom performed because of technical difficulties.

Probable Alzheimer's disease is diagnosed when there are typical clinical features and the many other causes of dementia have been ruled out by investigation. Possible Alzheimer's disease is diagnosed when there are atypical features present or where there are additional disorders that might account for some of the symptoms. Thus the common idea that Alzheimer's disease can be diagnosed on an either/or basis like measles, is seen to be totally erroneous.

I have dealt with this disease in some detail only because it is so prevalent in later life, so much in the news and so widely feared. There are many other organic causes of dementia which I will not deal with; they are a matter for your doctor.

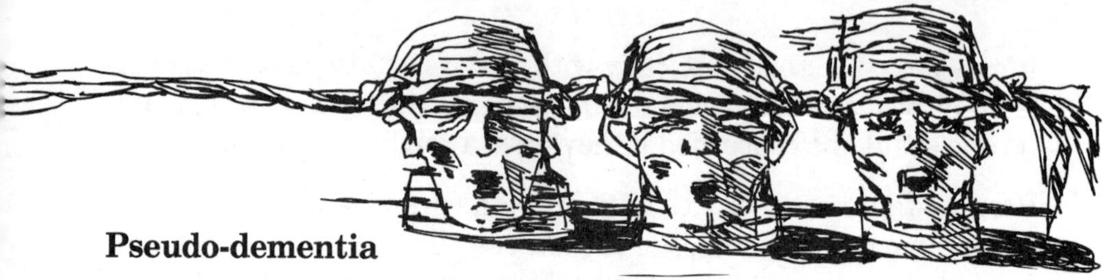

Pseudo-dementia

There are many functional (psychological) disorders that may be mistaken for true dementia of the organic variety. There are 101 reasons why a person might appear to be losing his or her memory and general competence. Chief among them are various types of depression, and someone with an organic state may develop a functional disorder in addition. The important thing about pseudo-dementia is that the condition may clear up completely, and the patient return to normal when the circumstances of life improve.

The dangers of amateur diagnosis

Alzheimer's disease is one of these conditions that are widespread and greatly feared, like cancer, and it is difficult to establish whether it is or is not present in many cases. It has therefore been the subject of much amateur speculation, and some really weird therapies have been proposed. People who fear that they may be suffering from it because they are becoming rather forgetful (say, because they are worried and depressed) may resort to one of these amateur therapies, and if their psychological state improves with changing circumstances, they may then imagine that they have cured themselves of Alzheimer's disease by swallowing the 'snake oil' they obtained at a high price from some sort of medicine man – and tell their friends so! You should beware of the ill-written books that are published by people who have no relevant qualifications.

If you are concerned in any way about Alzheimer's disease you should get in touch with the Alzheimer's Disease Society, the address of which is given in Appendix A.

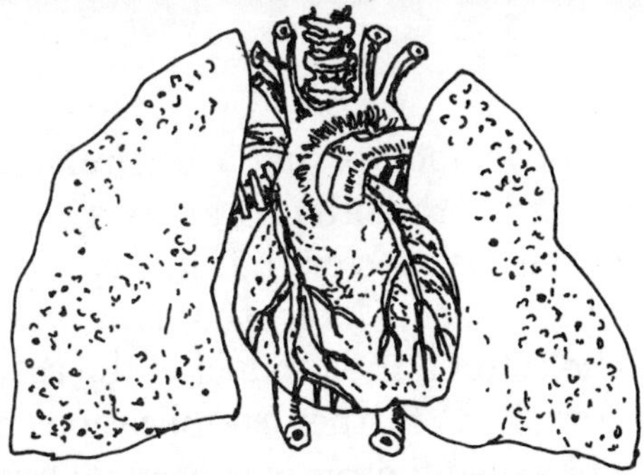

ISCHAEMIC HEART DISEASE

In ischaemic heart disease the passageways through the arteries that supply the heart muscle with blood become narrowed. The disorder takes place in two phases: first, there are atheromatous deposits ('gunge' as previously described) accumulating within the arteries without any symptoms becoming noticeable; second, some of this matter may become detached and cause blockages so that the heart muscle is starved of blood. The result is acute pain and some of the heart muscle may die. The good news is that the damaged muscle has remarkable properties of re-growth, and some individuals may have repeated attacks over a long span of years and yet survive, living quite active lives into a ripe old age.

The disease poses many problems that have not yet been understood. There are wide variations in its incidence between different countries: for instance, Japan has less than 80 deaths per 100,000 of the population annually, compared with over 400 in both Scotland and Northern Ireland, with England and Wales coming close behind. Immediately we think of the very dissimilar diet of the Japanese, with fish dishes replacing most of our meat, and a high intake of rice. But if we look at the 13 countries for which figures are given in a Royal College of Physicians publication, France and Italy come close behind Japan, and I have never noticed our continental cousins stinting themselves of meat, fatty cheeses and butter. Aha, we think, it is all the wine the French and Italians drink that protects them – perhaps this is the case – but I see that Hungary comes very close to the British figures for heart disease, and I buy plenty of Hungarian wine.

The truth seems to be that heart disease is caused by many

complex factors that are unrelated to one another, and are connected with both diet and way of life. In the UK smoking is a strong risk factor, but in Japan it has no relation to the disease, thus it seems likely that only when the blood has a high level of cholesterol, the product of the saturated fats, will smoking cause trouble. A further complication that is apparent from the published figures is that in all countries listed the rates for men are very much higher than for women. Everywhere men and women eat much the same, but they do not behave the same – is this a significant clue?

We must not forget the curious results of Grossarth-Maticek which were displayed earlier on page 179, (which some commentators dismiss as being too good to be true) that imply that there is a very strong link between heart-attacks and Type A behaviour. As well as the two sexes differing in behaviour, they differ in physiology. Older women should note that after the age of menopause the rates for women and men converge, and it may be that hormone replacement therapy will have a protective effect.

Out of all this morass of complex data what do the experts advise older people to do to lessen the risk of heart disease which is the main cause of death for older men and second only to cancer among women? They are not very optimistic about preventive measures for it seems that the disorder has its roots in factors in middle-age and even in childhood.

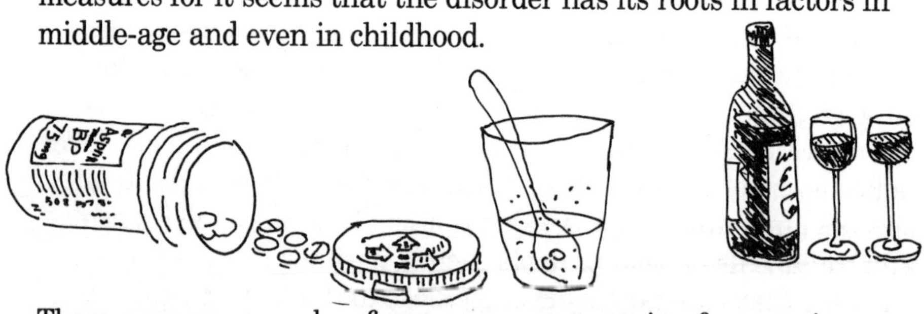

There are some crumbs of encouragement coming from various recent research studies: I have already mentioned the good news about drinking wine, and it would be wonderful if in the next budget there were a provision for pensioners getting a reduction at off-licenses (it might save the NHS some money!) Recent work has shown that a small daily dose of aspirin combined with certain other drugs, may reduce further heart-attacks by as much as 25 to 40%, so that is good news for the not inconsiderable number of older people who have already had a warning attack.

In general, the advice is simply following the principles that have already been discussed in earlier chapters – sensible diet, adequate exercise, controlling your Type A behaviour, enjoying what you most fancy in a moderate manner, and what you save on cigarettes may be spent on a little extra wine with safety.

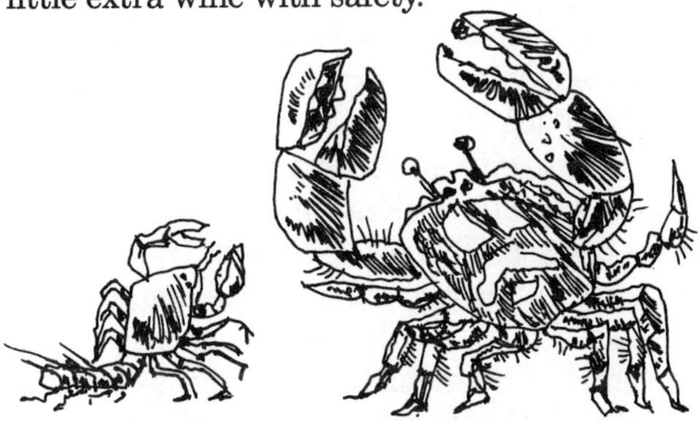

CANCERS

In the Western world cancer is predominantly a disease of later life, and over half of the cases occur over the age of 65. It is a somewhat mysterious disease in that although there is an obvious connection between some cancers and environmental irritants such as tobacco smoke and lung cancer, and prolonged exposure to strong sunlight and skin cancer, why it develops in one part of the body rather than another in most individuals is unknown. It seems likely that the individual has a vulnerability that is local, and the environmental irritant triggers the pathological process. This vulnerability may be genetically determined in some cases: for instance, although tobacco smoke is an established risk factor it is specially likely to affect the lungs of 10% of individuals with a particular genetic constitution.

The sort of life that people lead, including their diet and occupation, is obviously related to the kind of cancers they develop. Thus in Japan there is a high prevalence of stomach cancer, but when Japanese immigrants to America have lived there for a generation or so, the incidence of stomach cancer decreases, but that of breast cancer increases to a rate similar to that of the native Americans. Although it has been established at what anatomical sites cancers typically strike in different countries, it is difficult to say why, as there are so many environmental hazards interacting with the genetic predispositions of the people of those countries.

It has long been suspected that vulnerability to cancer is partly determined by the personality of the individual and hence the type of life he or she leads. If this was confirmed and clarified it would be possible to give advice to people at risk of cancer, particularly in later life when the risk is high, so that they might avoid developing the disease. The researches of Grossarth-Maticek and his colleagues in Yugoslavia have been mentioned, but these results have been received with a good deal of scepticism. One medical commentator, referring to the analysis of the results, remarked that if this had been a better analysis:

> it would have contributed to the credibility of their message that risk of cancer and CHD can be greatly diminished, and that duration of survival may be increased by psychological treatment . . . If it were possible to diminish the risk of cancer and CHD and to increase duration of survival in these ways, "what a wonderful world it would be".

Needless to say these criticisms have been answered and the controversy continues in the manner of most disputes between scientists which are fairly incomprehensible to the lay public.

The following advice about minimizing the risk of developing cancer is broadly agreed on by doctors today, with only a little controversy surrounding it. Take action to avoid the following risks:

1. **Smoking is associated with cancer of the lungs and probably some other organs.**
2. **Prolonged exposure to strong sunlight may cause cancer of the skin.**
3. **Frequent contact with some irritant chemicals may also cause skin cancer.**
4. **Sexual promiscuity in both male and female is associated with cancer of the cervix.**
5. **Excessive alcohol intake may damage the liver and lead to cancer of that organ.**

It is evident that there are only a few actual steps that you can take to avoid some manifestations of cancer in later life, but a lot can be done in the way of monitoring your health to ensure that some early signs do not go unnoticed.

Unexplained and long-continued tiredness, poor appetite, loss of weight, change in bowel function, development of 'bumps' in any part of the body, may all be indicative of developing cancer and should be reported to your doctor for medical investigation. These signs may have a perfectly innocuous meaning, and even actual growths may be 'benign', but without becoming a hypochondriac it is better to be safe than sorry, and many forms of cancer can be eradicated if they are diagnosed early.

According to Age Concern:

> Breast screening, in terms of lives saved for each screening, is thought even more effective in women aged 65 - 74 (more research is needed on women of 75+) than in younger women . . . If you are 65 or over you will not be invited for breast screening, but you are entitled to NHS screening on request every three years.

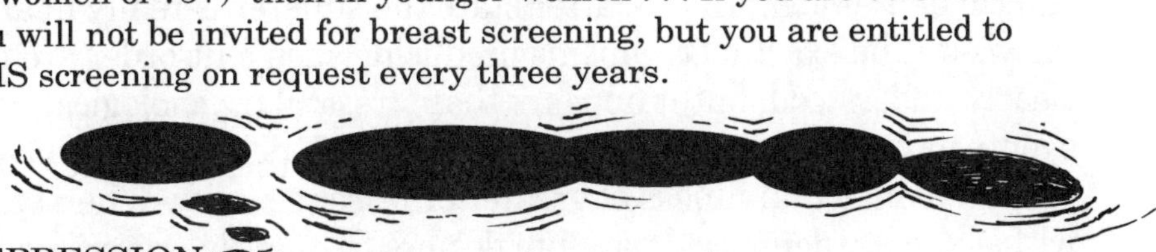

DEPRESSION

It used to be held that 'depression' was the natural accompaniment of growing old. This attitude has now been abandoned, and one medical writer, having reviewed all the many stressful factors that older people have to cope with in contemporary society, asked the question ' Why is not every old person in a profound state of depression?'

You will note that I have put the word 'depression' in inverted commas; this is because there are various criteria for depression among health professionals. Some experts on the subject suggest that 1 in 10 of 'the elderly population' (presumably those over statutory retirement age) can be diagnosed as being depressed, while others estimate that the proportion is 1 in 4. Obviously they are using quite different criteria. Psychiatrists used to contrast 'reactive' with 'endogenous' depression, the latter term implying that the more serious condition had arisen from some basic disorder of the brain chemistry in contrast to just a strong reaction to on-going circumstances; now it is more usual to refer to the milder reactive form as 'dysthymia' and the more serious form as 'major depression'. In this chapter I am concerned with the milder and more common forms of depression, and so in order to discuss the matter I must make clear what I mean by the term.

All normal people know what it feels like to be a bit depressed at times, and may refer to the state as being down in the dumps, thoroughly fed up, afflicted by the black dog, and similar expressions denoting a low mood, but there is a definite difference between a temporary condition of mental dejection and being in a state of clinical depression. In the latter state the sufferer is really ill and knows it. The exact mechanisms producing such a disorder are not clearly understood, but it appears that stressful psychological events have altered the chemical processes of the brain and have produced an actual illness of greater or lesser severity. When faced with clinically depressed patients doctors frequently prescribe anti-depressant drugs the purpose of which is to re-adjust the brain chemistry. Drug treatment for depression is a huge area of medical and psychological debate, and unfortunately these drugs, which now exist in a wide variety of forms, sometimes have no beneficial effect whatsoever.

When normally down in the dumps we can generally be cheered up by a pleasant event or an enlivening companion, but clinically depressed people are depressed for 24 hours in the day with little variation and do not react to normally cheering events. The results of depression are apathy, worry over trivia, inability to take pleasure in anything, and utter pessimism. Often there is severe insomnia and obsessive worry about the apparent malfunction of various body processes when there is nothing really wrong.

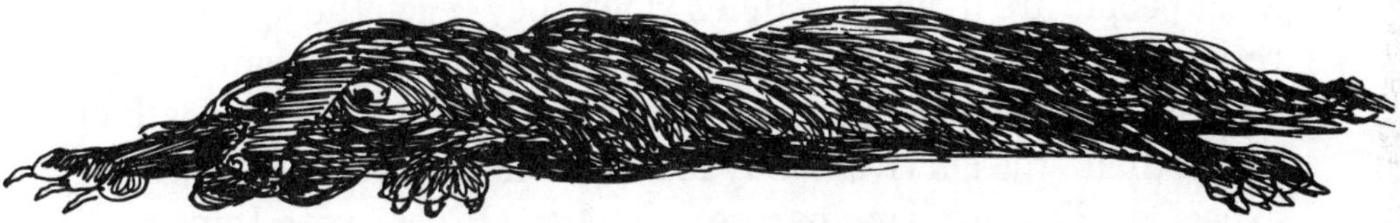

It can indeed be a serious illness, and when anti-depressant drugs do not work depressed patients may be hospitalized for electro-convulsive therapy. The latter has had a bad press and some are very hostile to it almost as a matter of principle, but in the experience of some doctors it is the treatment of choice for elderly people if they are deeply depressed. It does not 'cure' the depression, but it provides a respite in which the sufferer can set to and take positive action to re-organize his or her way of life.

Having attempted to define the nature of clinical depression, I shall now consider the risk factors and discuss how the risks of depression in later life may be minimized – for it is certainly not inevitable, and despite the inevitable pessimism of people in this condition, they have to accept the fact that they may recover completely and be their ordinary selves again. The main risk factors are events and conditions that rob the individual of the normal power to cope with the demands of the environment. Bereavement, sudden disability, loss of social status, loneliness, perceived economic deprivation, chronic pain, and above all a feeling of having no place in the world, are all hazards of growing old in the youth-oriented society in which we live, and powerful generators of depression.

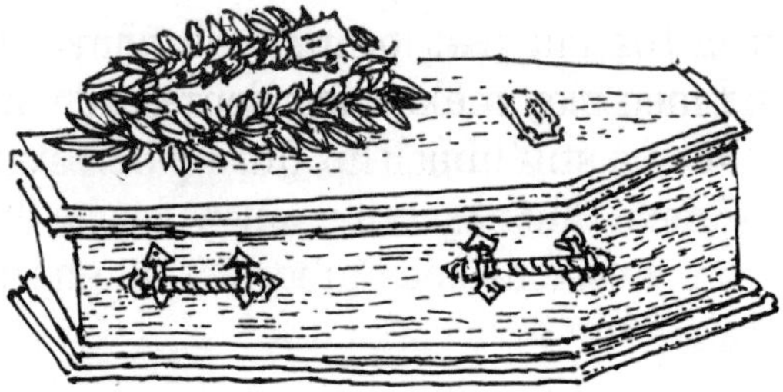

1. Bereavement

Most people are living in couples when they reach the age of retirement and although they may not feel very dependent on each other in the relationship, when it is dissolved through the death of one of them, the survivors may feel far more bereft than they expected. The surviving partner may have to cope with things that he or she never thought about before, and although it sounds shamefully mundane it is often trivial things that assume an overwhelming and disproportionate importance. Widowers tend to be harder hit than widows, and there is a raised incidence of death amongst men in the year following bereavement. The bereaved person may feel ashamed of some of the aspects of his or her deprivation; Wendy and Sally Greengross write of one aspect of bereavement that many people do not like to admit to, especially when they are of quite an advanced age:

> The pain of this overwhelming loss is often made worse because the surviving partner quite unexpectedly finds that he or she has sexual feelings that demand satisfaction. Some of the need may be for touching, comfort or caring, but some people still have strong physical sexual desires. These create confusion for those for whom it is still a struggle to find emotional stability, and the lack of open discussion

arouses fear that no-one else has such feelings or desires. The conspiracy of silence that society imposes on this topic often prevents widows and widowers seeking appropriate advice and reassurance.

There is a sense of loss that is difficult to describe; some writers have referred to it as 'lack of a confiding relationship' and it is important in the generation of a depressed state. Women are rather better than men at forming 'confiding relationships' in our society, and men may make their depressed state worse by endeavouring to 'keep a stiff upper lip' during bereavement. There is a dreadful modern taboo on the mention and acknowledgement of death, and bereaved people tend to be boycotted by friends and acquaintances who simply don't know how to behave in the situation. Their unexpected withdrawal of social support makes the widow or widower feel additionally alone.

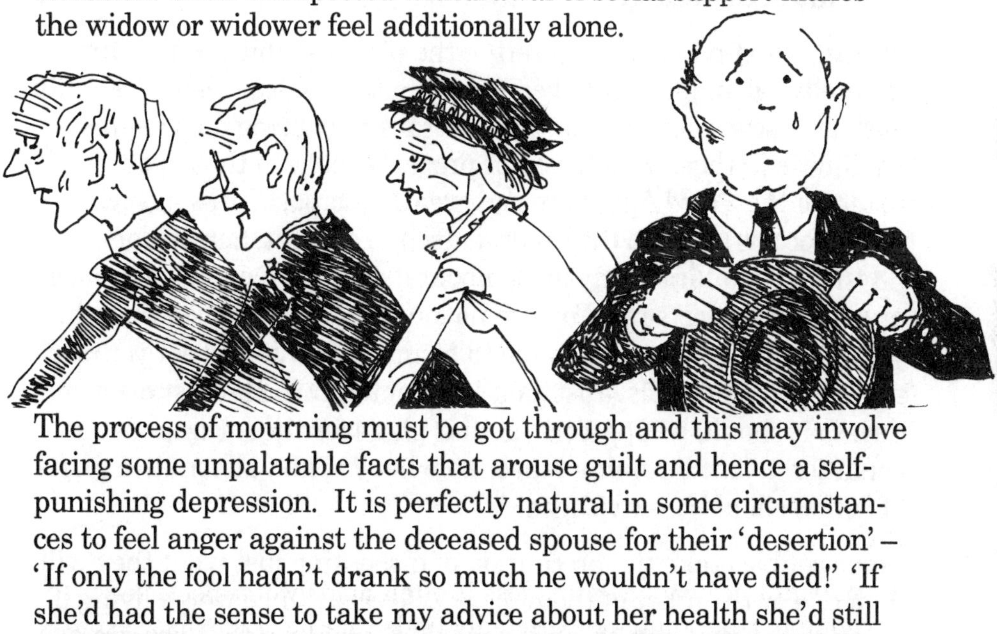

The process of mourning must be got through and this may involve facing some unpalatable facts that arouse guilt and hence a self-punishing depression. It is perfectly natural in some circumstances to feel anger against the deceased spouse for their 'desertion' – 'If only the fool hadn't drank so much he wouldn't have died!' 'If she'd had the sense to take my advice about her health she'd still be here!' It is also natural to feel a sense of *relief* that the loved one has died, especially when there has been a long illness that has been stressful for the carer. These feelings about one's own selfishness and human weakness should be frankly acknowledged during the mourning process, as well as the remorse that can be summed up as, 'If only I'd been a more caring wife/husband maybe he/she would be alive today.' Depression generally has a component of self-punishing guilt that can only be got rid of by consciously admitting reality rather than shrouding the whole matter of bereavement in conventional platitudes.

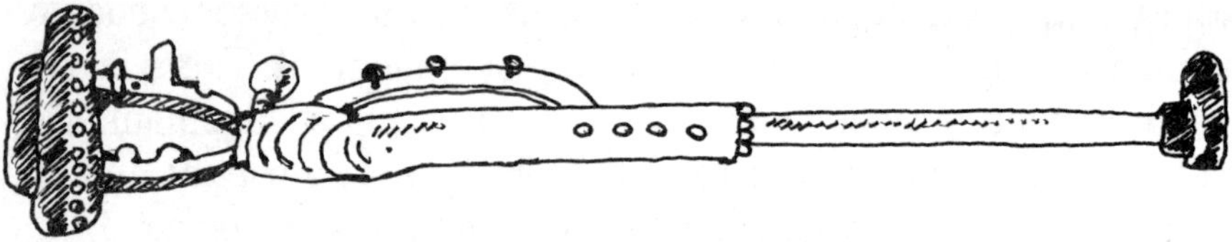

2. Sudden disability

Suddenly to find yourself bereft of the physical abilities that are normally taken for granted can be a shattering experience. Events such as a severe heart-attack or a stroke may bring on a depressive illness in those who have not properly realized that upon entering the Third Age there is a greatly increased risk of such events occurring. Or, the gradual decline of sight, hearing or physical capabilities may bring about a change in one's self image or a loss of self esteem. You are no longer the person you thought you were and you need to come to terms with this and set yourself new, achievable goals. Just as it is accepted that all must die some day, so it should be appreciated that plans for the future must be conditional on continuing reasonable health, and alternative plans of action should be envisaged.

Some couples take the precaution of discussing just what they will do if one or the other of them dies. Life can still be worth living if a crippling event occurs, and it should be realized that you are just lucky if the Third Age can be lived through in a state of fair health and mobility with a living partner. While enjoying the present you should have the vision to anticipate several possible futures.

3. Loss of social status

People sometimes succumb to depression after retirement if they have been very dependent for their self-image on the position they have occupied in the world of work. Note the way *Mastermind* contestants invariably identify themselves as a retired this or that. To have been a head of department or other important figure in some organization may mean far too much to some individuals, and they may have neglected to develop interests outside their sphere of work.

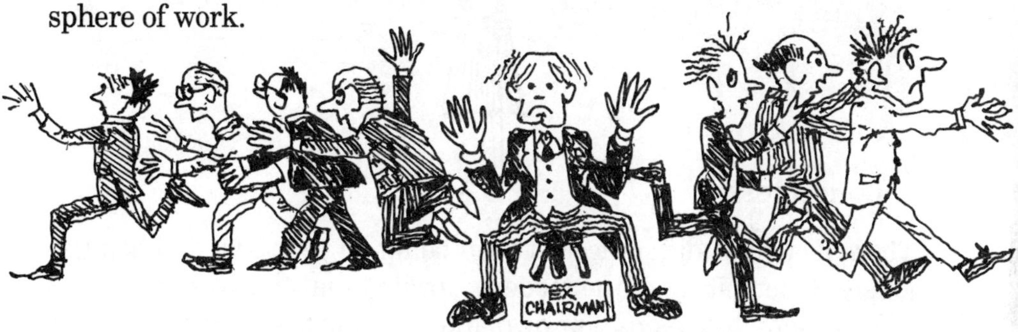

Our society is not kind to older people and this applies even within families. A man may have been a respected paterfamilias, but children grow up and develop their own interests and values which may be very different from those of their parents, so father may find rather suddenly that no-one pays any attention to his opinions any more and that he is rather unwanted at family gatherings because he still expects to throw his weight around. The same may apply to mothers who used to be so useful as baby-sitters for the young grandchildren, but if she becomes unable to cope with small children or when these become independent teenagers she may find the family distinctly ungrateful, and offer her no role at all to fulfil.

It is therefore a great mistake for parents to invest too much in the lives of their middle-aged offspring whose attitudes and behaviour may be determined by pressures of which the older generation knows very little; rather, grandparents should build up worthwhile lives for themselves and aim at self-fulfilment in the Third Age independently of the concerns of the younger generation. If they continue to have close ties with their families – fine, but they should not count on it, for a sense of rejection engenders depression.

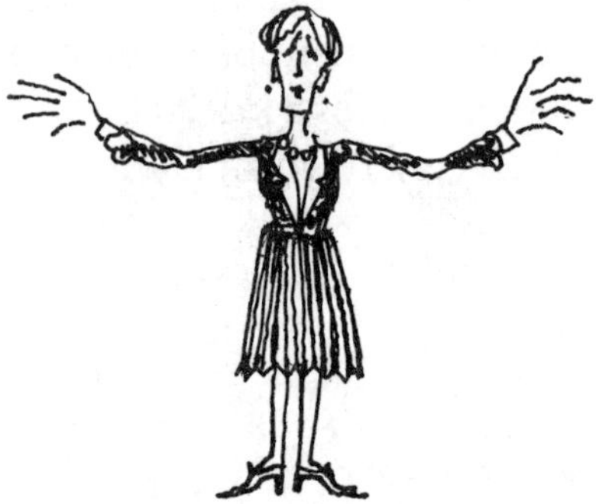

4. Loneliness

There is a great difference between being on your own and being lonely. One feature of the modern world is that there are many older women living on their own and enjoying their freedom from a previous life of domestic responsibility and catering for the needs of husbands and children. Widowhood or divorce does not necessarily lead to loneliness, but it can. Loneliness is being on your own when you would rather have the company of other people, not just to sit with as you might in a pub, but to be involved with in some common purpose.

In the UK about 35% of retired people live on their own and 52% with only their spouse who is generally elderly also. It is possible, of course, to be lonely whilst living in the company of someone else, when neither partner shares the same interests or has activities in common. Work, particularly when it is shared with other people, is an excellent antidote to depression. The whole concept of retirement is coming under scrutiny; it is fine for those who have absorbing interests to occupy their new leisure time, but not everyone has such interests and may have relied on the company of their workmates to give them a sense of community; the cessation of work may contribute to the development of loneliness and hence depression. Fortunately there are many avenues for voluntary work after retirement, and new interests and new friends can be acquired in the Third Age.

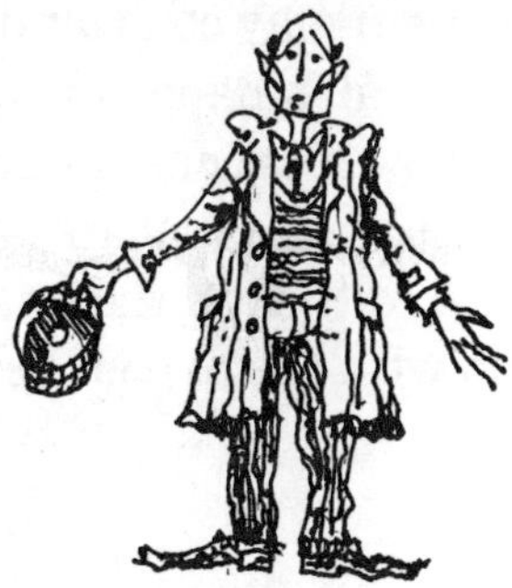

5. Perceived economic deprivation

I say 'perceived' economic deprivation for it is your perception of poverty rather than its actuality that is more likely to lead to a condition of depression. I do not suggest that people should be content to live on a pittance having worked all their lives in a society that wastes so much wealth, but those who have every reason to be discontented with their lot are not necessarily depressed.

The healthy reaction is to kick against the pricks and try to do something about it, for as long as you are angry and kicking, you will not succumb to depression. It is the slide into apathy and the 'slough of despond' that has pathological consequences. People may be quite reasonably well off by contemporary standards, but if they have been accustomed to a much higher standard of living, and in later life perceive themselves to be wretchedly impoverished and helpless then they are very vulnerable indeed.

6. Chronic pain.

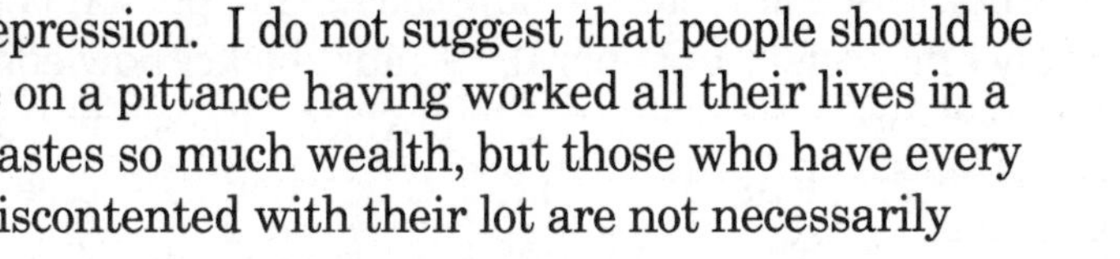

There is a strong relationship between depression and chronic pain. The latter term is often applied to conditions in which no physical cause can be found for the persistent pain; there may once have been a wound which has healed completely, and it seems as if the pain is in the mind, a memory of a past pain that will not go away. In such cases the pain may come and go according to the mental state of the individual; a happy event such as falling in love and forming a good new relationship may bring someone out of the depression and the pain disappears. Just treating the pain with drugs will not cure it, although the original painful condition may have had a lot to do with the person becoming depressed in the first place.

Summary

A lot of space has been given to discussion of depression because unlike the types of disability in later life that were mentioned earlier, it is not directly linked to the age-related weakening of the body but to social factors – how the ageing person is treated by the family and society in general. It must be acknowledged, of course, that as depression is related to physical illness, we are at greater risk in later life as far as that is concerned. To some extent depression is preventable and curable, but the steps to be taken are not wholly within the power of the sufferer, although he or she can do a lot in the way of self-help if the causes of the disorder are understood.

Individuals vary greatly in their tendency to become depressed, and those who react to adverse influences in later life by developing such a disorder may have had depressive episodes when they were younger. In more recent years clinical psychologists have developed techniques for treating the milder forms of depression by what is known as 'psychological therapy', and this may be very effective.

The generations that are now entering the Third Age differ from those who went before them in that they are better able to stand up for themselves and less willing to accept an inferior status in society because they are 'old'. It may follow that the incidence of depression in later life will get less as time progresses, although some would argue that as society increases in its complexity we will have more difficult challenges to meet!

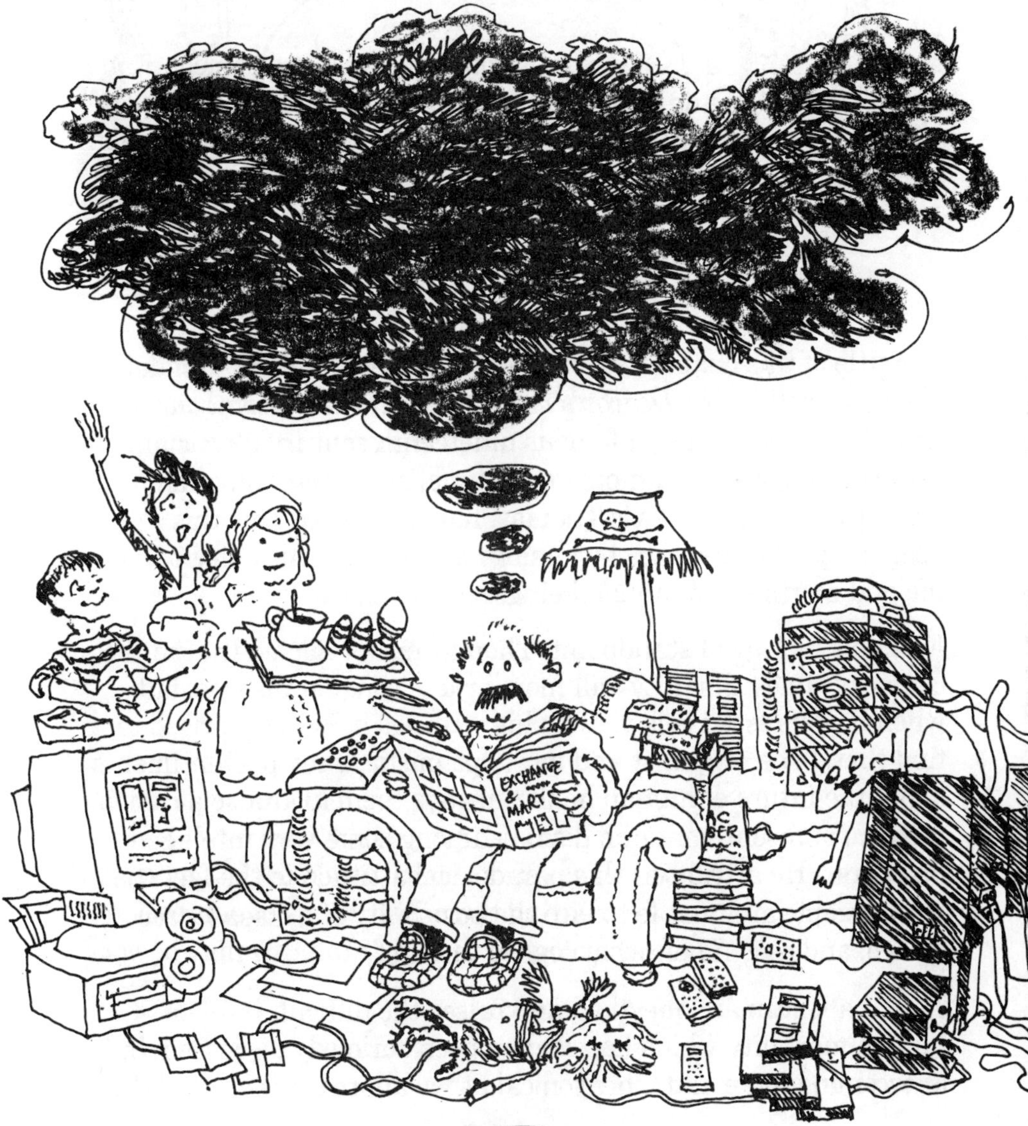

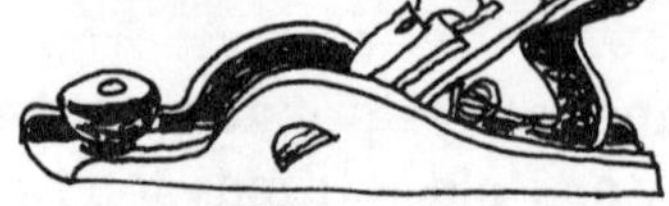

Chapter 9

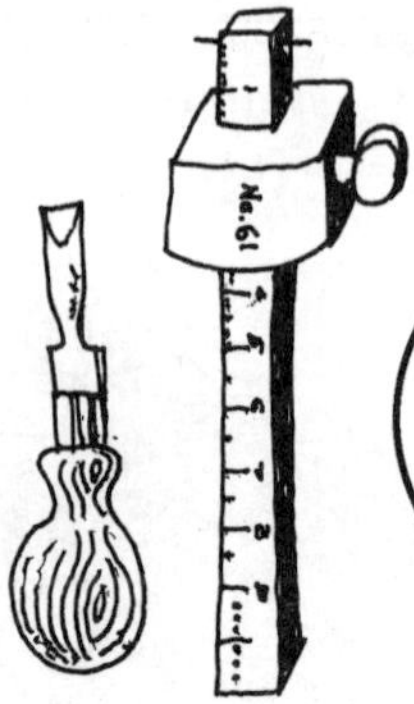

THE ONE-HOSS SHAY

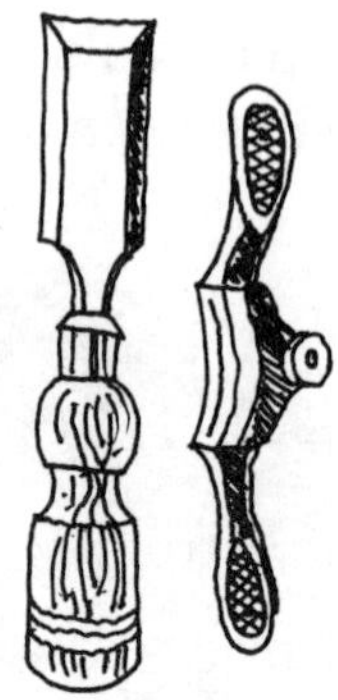

The title of this chapter refers to some verses by Oliver Wendell Holmes entitled *The Deacon's masterpiece: the wonderful one-hoss shay.* Wendell Holmes, a famous nineteenth century physician, wit and essayist, was a man before his time, and a contemporary American biologist, Lewis Thomas, has recognized how this doggerel poem expresses by analogy a profound truth about the life and mortality of human beings.

From his biological standpoint, Thomas has predicted that in the course of time humanity will more or less conquer disease, but when he expressed this view in his writings he was surprised to find that, 'The brightest and most optimistic of my presentiments about the future of human health always seem to arouse a curious mixture of resentment and dismay among some very intelligent listeners.' He attributes this paradoxical attitude to the fact that many people are unable to face the possibility of a disease-free future, and ask, 'Then what are we to die of?'

This is a legitimate question, and raises the difficult issue of human mortality which has seldom been seriously discussed, but is becoming more and more topical as we approach the possibility of the conquest of disease. In seeking an answer Thomas harks back to Oliver Wendell Holmes and his doggerel tale of the wonderful one-hoss shay which he recognizes as a brilliant analogy. The verses tell the story of how the Deacon planned and built a wonderful horse-drawn vehicle with durability and longevity in mind. It begins:

Have you heard of the wonderful one-hoss shay,

That was built in such a logical way

It ran for a hundred years to a day,

And then, of a sudden, it — ah but stay,

I'll tell you what happened without delay,

Scaring the parson into fits,

Frightening people out of their wits —

Have you ever heard of that, I say?

It goes on to describe how the Deacon chose the materials for every component of the shay he was building with the utmost care:

So the Deacon inquired of the village folk

Where he could find the strongest oak,

That couldn't be split nor bent nor broke

The problem was that in any such machine as a horse-drawn shay wear and tear would eventually find out the weakest spot and hence it would break down and require constant mending and patching up before eventually becoming a wreck, and the Deacon attempted to avoid this by the care he took in designing the vehicle and the use of excellent materials in construction:

But the Deacon swore (as Deacons do,

With an 'I dew vum' or an 'I tell yeou')

He would build one shay to beat the town

''N the keounty 'n' all the kentry roun':

It should be so built that it couldn't break down.

Two American professors, James Fries and Lawrence Crapo, specialists in geriatric medicine at Stanford University, have followed Lewis Thomas and used the tale as an analogy to illustrate their remarkable theory of ageing which is set out in their book *Vitality and Aging*. They write:

The myths of the super-centenarian, of Shangri-la, and of Methuselah crumble upon close examination. Yet in the rubble, we find hope for a meaningful rejuvenation – where the maximum lifespan is not prolonged but the period of vitality is.

If we human beings were perfectly designed and free from all diseases then, as many people have dreamed, we would never break down and live for ever. This dream has existed since ancient times and is based upon three myths: the Hyperborean myth concerning special places where the inhabitants live to a phenomenal age, the myth of the supercentenarians, the myth of the Fountain of Youth.

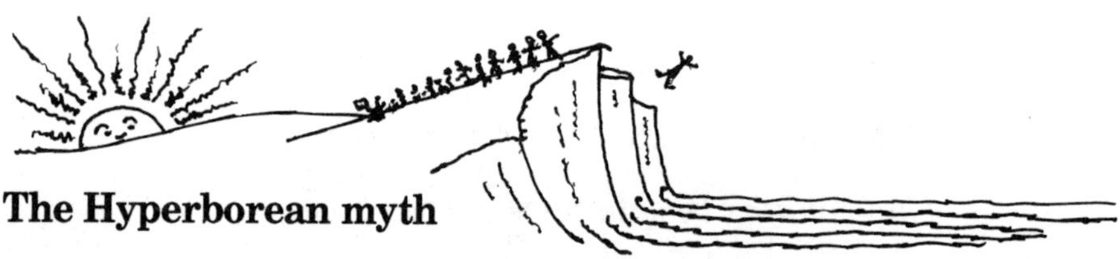

The Hyperborean myth

This is a Greek myth of a land existing 'beyond the north wind' where there was perpetual sunshine and whose inhabitants lived in continuous peace and harmony with perfect health. The length of their lives was normally 1,000 years, but if anyone became tired of life he would dress in ceremonial regalia and leap off a cliff into the sea. Versions of this myth occur in the folk-lore of many cultures. More recently James Hilton published a novel, *Lost Horizon*, which centres on a remote region of the Himalayas, Shangri-La, where the people lived ideal lives like the mythical Hyperboreans and attained extreme longevity.

In the 1960s researchers into longevity wondered whether there were, in fact, remote regions of the world where remarkably long lives were attained and they set out to discover them, reasoning that they might learn important facts about diet and life-style which would be useful in guiding our behaviour in the more developed countries. For a time the prospect seemed rosy, and all sorts of good advice was publicized concerning how we might emulate these primitive people, but the researchers eventually found that they had been misled as to the longevity in these places.

It is all very well to live an unstressful life in the pure air of remote mountainous regions, to drink little or no alcohol, and not to smoke cigarettes, but what you gain on the swings thereby you are apt to lose on the roundabouts, for these people were denied the benefits of modern medicine and public hygiene, and on balance these alleged Hyperboreans might have a lower expectancy of life than is found in the more developed nations.

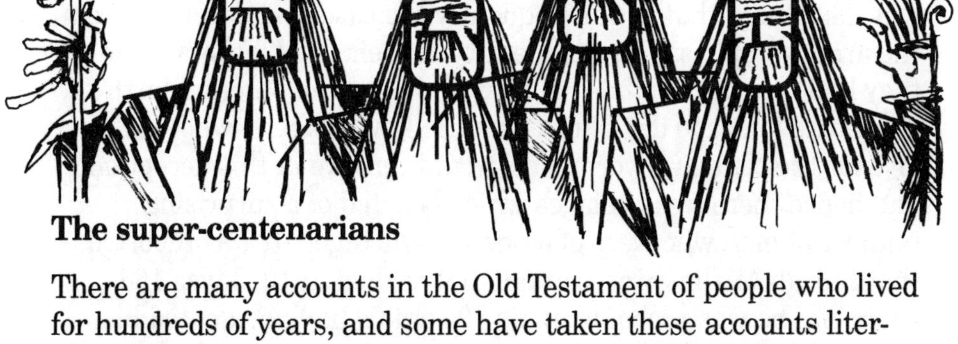

The super-centenarians

There are many accounts in the Old Testament of people who lived for hundreds of years, and some have taken these accounts literally, believing that such super-centenarians actually had such incredibly long lives in ancient times.

As mentioned previously, earlier in this century reports began to accumulate about populations in different parts of the world where many people lived to a very great age and retained their vigour to a far greater extent than is normal in the advanced Western nations. Among the populations studied were those of the villages of Vilcamamba in Ecuador, the Hunza in Kashmir, and Abkhazia in the USSR, where it was reputed that many people lived to a great age. It was claimed that some common denominators of extreme longevity had been discovered, including no retirement from work, a moderate indulgence in 'vices', a strong sex-drive, fertility in women, and limited calorific intake.

Later inquiries have thrown doubt on the information that the people themselves gave to those questioning them, and the researchers eventually realized that they had been misled in Ecuador. It is difficult to conduct such inquiries in places where the registration of births a long time ago was not very accurate, and where the people themselves, proud of their reputation, have a motive for exaggerating their age. Various researchers have thrown doubt on the validity of the early findings; it was eventually discovered that the supposedly long-lived Ecuadorians actually have a life expectancy less than that of the population of the USA. As for the supposedly long-lived men of South Russia, it was discovered that it was frequently the case that deserters from the army would assume the identity of their dead fathers when they had returned to their villages and used the parental birth certificate to evade detection. Their fellow villagers, who had no love for the central government, would connive at this deception and hence there were villages which boasted of a surprising number of men who were of a phenomenal age. It was reported that Shirali Mislimov of Azerbaijan who died in 1973 was 168 years old; he was probably in his 80s or 90s having adopted his father's birth certificate when younger and subsequently destroyed it as there were no written records of his age at the time of his death. The *1980 Guinness Book of World Records* accepts as documented only five persons living beyond the age of 112 years, the oldest being Shigechiyo Isumi in Japan who lived for 114 years. More recently there has been a report of a woman in France living to the age of 120 years.

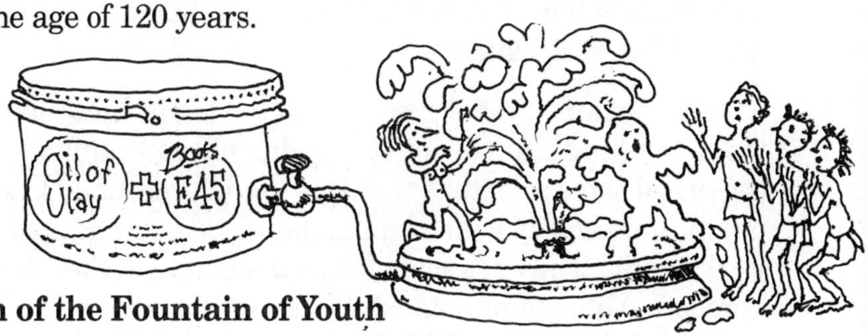

The myth of the Fountain of Youth

The myth of there being a magical Fountain of Youth has occurred in various cultures for centuries, and it has taken different forms. This fountain was supposed to cure all ills and to confer eternal youth on those who bathed in it. The Renaissance artist Lucas Cranach used it for the subject of a painting in which wrinkled elderly women plunge into the water at one side, while others are emerging at the other rejuvenated, to be greeted by a band of expectant young men, thus illustrating the sexual theme that partly fuels the yearning for rejuvenation. Modern manufacturers of cosmetics go some way to creating this fantasy of wishful thinking in their advertisements for their products.

The 16th Century Portuguese adventurer Ponce de Leon believed that such a fountain existed in the fabled land of 'Bimini', which he had been told of by the Indians of Puerto Rico, and set out with three ships to find it. What de Leon actually discovered was Florida and was made Governor of it by his King.

The search for the Fountain of Youth has been associated with a belief that longevity is in some way connected with sexuality, and many of the ancient nostrums that were supposed to promote longevity contained material from the sexual organs of animals. One of the first attempts to prolong life and rejuvenate men in terms of modern medicine was that of Charles Brown-Sequard who injected himself with testicular material from various animals and claimed that it had produced in him renewed vigour and enjoyment of life. This was in 1889 when he was 72 years of age; he died five years later.

Experiments in various species with the transplantation of the testes of young animals into the bodies of senile animals, convinced some scientists that this would eventually lead to a practical means by which human life could be prolonged. Such work is principally associated with the names of Steinach and Voronoff. Voronoff implanted the testes of monkeys in elderly men and claimed that this did indeed rejuvenate them, but as the experiments were not properly controlled, there was no evidence that it had any effect on their life-span. From what we now know about organ implantation, and the actual effects of the injection of testosterone, it is plain that Voronoff's experiments could have had no relevant physiological effect on his patients, but their status was probably improved by the placebo effect.

Quite recently the Fountain of Youth myth resurfaced in reports that the drug Gerovital had miraculous powers of prolonging life, and the media eagerly seized on stories that various powerful world figures were being rejuvenated by it: stories that were soon to be denied by the death of these figures. Vitamin E is also credited with the power of rejuvenating and restoring sexual potency to men: a hardy chestnut that is repeatedly being denied in the scientific literature.

It should be noted that the Fountain myth has two aspects to it, one of greatly prolonging life and the other of conferring continued youthfulness. There is, of course, no point in living longer unless continued health and vigour are guaranteed as the Greek myth of Tithonus emphasises. Eos, goddess of the dawn, loved Tithonus, a mortal man, so she petitioned Zeus that he might live forever. The plea was granted, but she had not asked for his continued youthfulness, so while she retained her rosy beauty her lover withered as he aged. In Tennyson's poem based on the legend, he has Tithonus say:

Let me go: take back thy gift:

Why should a man desire in any way

To vary from the kindly race of men,

Or pass beyond the goal of ordinance

Where all should pause, as is most meet for all.

THE INVENTION OF DEATH

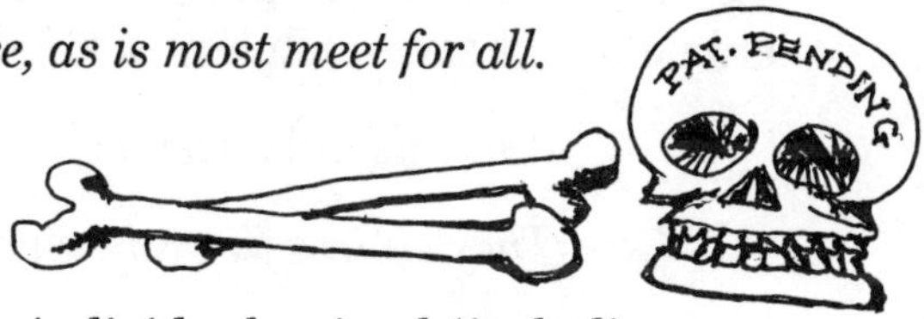

We take it for granted that every individual animal (including human beings) will have to die some day however healthy a life has been led. It is also known that different species of animals have a definite lifespan that cannot be extended beyond a maximum limit however favourable the conditions of life. Comparison between the different life-spans of some common species is shown in the following table:

PROBABLE LIFE-SPAN IN VARIOUS SPECIES

Galapagos tortoise	175 years	Rhesus monkey	29
Man	95 (?)	Cat	25
Horse	46	Kangaroo	16
Gorilla	40	Mink	10
Grizzly bear	31	Mouse	4

The figures in this table have been taken from various sources and are fairly tentative especially for species Man. A number of contemporary scientists have proposed various lengths of the life-span for the human species, even as long as 130 years, so I have put a query mark after 95 years. Obviously some exceptional individuals will live beyond the stated span, and there are men and women alive today who are well over 100 years old. The purpose of the table is to exemplify the fact that there are very great differences indeed between the different species even when they live in optimum conditions for their health.

The puzzle is, what determines the life-span of the different species? Obviously it has something to do with the size of the animal, as the larger animals tend to have the longer lives, but why does the human species live so much longer than many animals that are much larger? A demotic rhyme has it that:

Animals are strictly dry;

They sinless live and swiftly die;

But sinful, ginfull rum-soaked men

Survive for threescore years and ten.

This rhyme rather contradicts the biblical saying that 'The wages of sin is death'.

It may come as a surprise to learn that a certain class of creatures do not have any pre-determined life-span and are in fact immortal. There was a time in the evolution of life upon this planet when all living creatures were of this class, and these immortals are with us yet; they originated in the far-distant time before death had been 'invented'. Creatures in this class are, in the main, neither wholly animal nor wholly plant; they are single-celled and known as protozoa. Typically they are free-swimming (active and animal-like) and green (by trapping energy from the sun they are very plant-like).

By referring to the protozoa as immortal I do not mean to imply that any individual cannot be killed; of course it can, and billions are being killed all the time, but they have no pre-determined life-span ending in death, as have the 'higher' multicelled organisms.

They reproduce themselves by simply splitting into two, and these two halves become independent creatures which ultimately split and repeat this indefinitely. As this process has been going on for countless ages, those specimens that are swimming in our ponds are literally millions of years old, although the substance of their bodies is being constantly renewed.

Death came into this world when sex was 'invented' – I mean death in the sense of an individual having a definite pre-determined life-course ending in inevitable termination. This truth is curiously expressed in the legend of Adam and Eve in the Garden of Eden, and it is extraordinary that the people who originated this legend had no knowledge of biology or evolutionary science.

According to the legend, Adam and Eve began as sex-less beings who were presumably intended to be immortal by their Creator for he told Adam:

> Of every tree in the garden thou mayest freely eat: But of the tree of knowledge of good and evil, thou shalt not eat of it: for in the day that thou eatest thereof thou shalt surely die.

When they had disobeyed and eaten of the tree of knowledge they became sexual beings and hence were condemned to a life of work, suffering and eventual death. Their Creator said to Adam:

Curst is the ground for thy sake;

In sorrow shalt thou eat of it all the days of thy life . . .

In the sweat of thy face shalt thou eat bread,

Till thou return unto the ground;

For out of it wast thou taken:

For dust thou art,

And unto dust shalt thou return.

So Adam's potential immortality came to an end and he was allotted a life-span ending in inevitable death. Eve was told the following by her Creator:

I will greatly multiply thy sorrow and thy conception;

In sorrow shalt thou bring forth children;

And thy desire shall be to thy husband,

And he shall rule over thee.

Thus in a highly poetic and allegorical form the facts about how sexual reproduction and death came into the world at some stage of evolution are told, for the latter follows from the former.

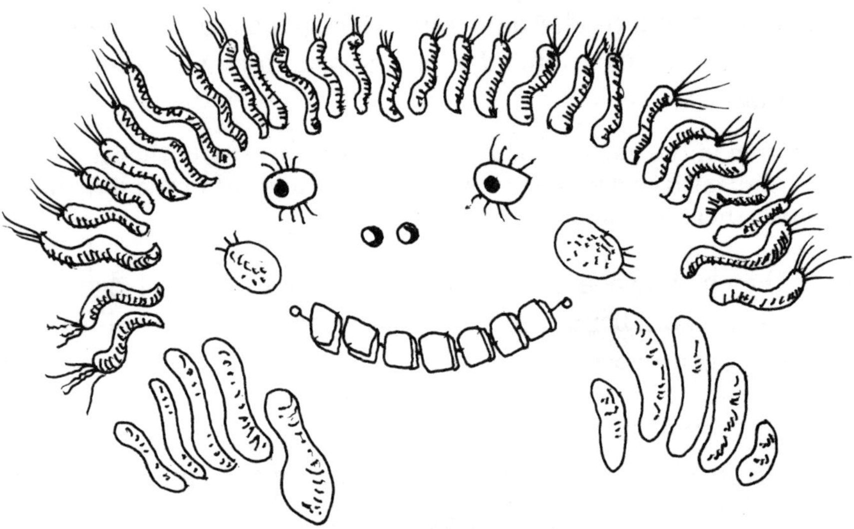

I began by referring to the one-celled organisms which are, in a sense, immortal and which reproduce simply by splitting. According to evolutionary theory these protozoa sometimes joined together to form multicellular units at some stage in the evolution of life, and when they did this the complex creatures which were thus formed evolved into the vast kingdom of animal and plant life on the planet. They share the common characteristic of consisting of co-operative colonies of cells specialized for different purposes.

Although some multicellular organisms can reproduce by splitting, just as you may take cuttings from a plant, they evolved a totally new form of reproduction which is sexual and typically involves the individual having a definite life-span and dying when the offspring have been produced.

I shall not go into the details of the genetics of sexual reproduction, and examine the evolutionary advantages that follow from this process; rather I will outline very roughly what takes place in its most primitive form. Some of the cells become specialized as sex cells of two varieties, male and female. In the most usual form, the male cells are active, free-swimming cells just like other protozoa, and they swim through water or other liquid media seeking the female cells. The latter are inert and swollen with food-reserves, sitting like Victorian maidens waiting for the arrival of a suitor who will penetrate them and mingle his genetic material with theirs.

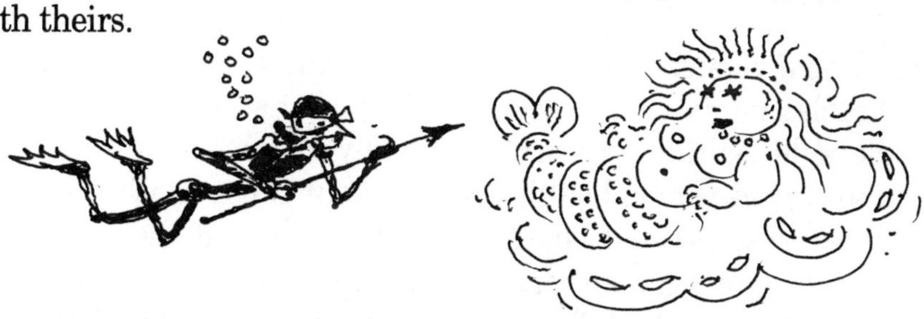

All this is well-known to schoolchildren nowadays when they study elementary biology, but what is less appreciated is the role that death has in this form of reproduction. Presumably it is of evolutionary advantage to a species for the parents to die when they have produced offspring, as otherwise they would clutter up the scene and compete for scarce resources with the younger generation who may have among them modified types of individuals more efficient than their parents in adapting to the ever-changing circumstances of the environment.

Here I shall quote from Joseph Krutch, who used the example of a primitive multicellular organism, Volvox, to illustrate how sexual reproduction led to a finite life-span ending with death. In his book *The Great Chain of Life* he has a chapter entitled very appropriately 'Enter love and enter death'. He relates how he has studied this tiny creature Volvox, green and just visible to the naked eye, which is commonly found in stagnant water. Like many primitive multicellular organisms that are partly animal and partly plant in their characteristics, it can reproduce both by budding and by sexual means. He writes:

> For Volvox, death seems to be as inevitable as it is in a mouse or in a man. Volvox must die as Leeuwenhoek saw it die because it has had children and is no longer needed. When its time comes it drops quietly to the bottom and joins its ancestors. As Hegner, the John Hopkins zoologist, once wrote,'This is the first advent of inevitable natural death in the animal kingdom and all for the sake of sex.' And as he asked, 'Is it worth it?' Nature's answer during all the years which have intervened between the first Volvox and quite recent times has been a pretty steady 'Yes'.

This long diversion into natural history makes clear why death is inevitable and natural to our species, and is not necessarily the result of ill-health. In theory, and ideally in practice, we should plan to stay in perfect health until the hour of our death. Our animal ancestors could expect to die just as soon as they became incapable of further reproduction, but one of the many ways in which human beings differ from simpler animals is that for us procreation is not just a matter of begetting children but involves many years of rearing them and of contributing to the welfare of the whole community in which they live long after these children have become independent.

For women the menopause marks the end of actually bearing children; in men there is no direct equivalent of the menopause and men can indeed remain fertile into advanced old age, but generally their sexuality broadens and becomes expressed in a wide field of creative activities.

Earlier in this book I have tried to define what is meant by the Third Age, a phenomenon that has become notable only in more recent times in the more advanced nations due to the practice of limiting family size, and the steady conquest of disease. People have generally referred to it in terms of the cessation of full-time employment whilst still perfectly fit, but it could equally well be referred to in terms of the 20 - 30 years of the life-span between the years of procreation, in its broadest sense, and death.

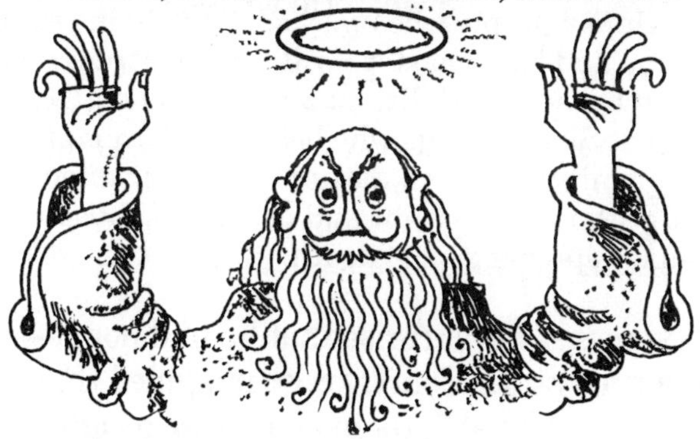

WOULD YOU LIKE TO BE IMMORTAL?

Some people have difficulty in accepting the fact that the day will come when they will no longer exist in this world, whatever beliefs they may have about a postulated after-life of the spirit. They may cherish the belief that if medical science were more advanced they would go on living far beyond their natural life-span. It is as if a mouse, whose life-span is given in the table above, were to aspire to live as long as a Galapagos tortoise if only his health were to improve! There is even a weird business of people paying to have their bodies kept in a frozen state after death so that they may be revivified when medical science has advanced so far that immortality is a practical possibility. Such a belief is based on a complete misunderstanding of health in relation to living. The mouse will never live for 175 years however healthy it may be because it is designed to have its limited little life-span and not that of a tortoise.

The question of the hankering for immortality was dealt with very effectively in the eighteenth century by Swift in *Gulliver's Travels*.

Gulliver visits the island of Luggnagg where he is told that they have people, known as Struldbruggs, who are immortal, and at first he is thrilled and excited by the idea of immortality and says:

> Happy nation where every child hath at least a chance for being immortal! Happy people who enjoy so many living examples of ancient virtue and have masters willing to instruct them in the wisdom of all former ages! But happiest beyond all comparison are these excellent Struldbruggs who being born exempt from that universal calamity of human nature have their minds free and disengaged without the weight and depression of spirits caused by the continual apprehension of death.

Gulliver expressed his surprise that he had not observed any of these immortals at the Court, for he imagined that the Prince would have had several of them about him as advisors and counsellors. When he had spoken in glowing terms of all the wonderful things he would do if he were granted immortality, the natives of the island disabused him of his illusions by showing him the Struldbruggs, some of them hundreds of years old, who exhibited all the disabilities and diseases of extreme old age, both physical and mental, including that of feeling socially isolated because they could not properly understand the contemporary language, 'thus they lie under the disadvantage of living like foreigners in their own country.'

Swift was, of course, confusing the diseases of later life (which must have been very serious in the eighteenth century) with age itself, but nevertheless he makes the point that we should aim to make the best of living in the social era in which we happen to be born, and not to hanker after continued life in an altered society that will become foreign to us.

THE SURVIVAL CURVE

In order to appreciate what has happened to the populations of the advanced nations in the present century during which the Third Age has developed, the following figure should be considered:

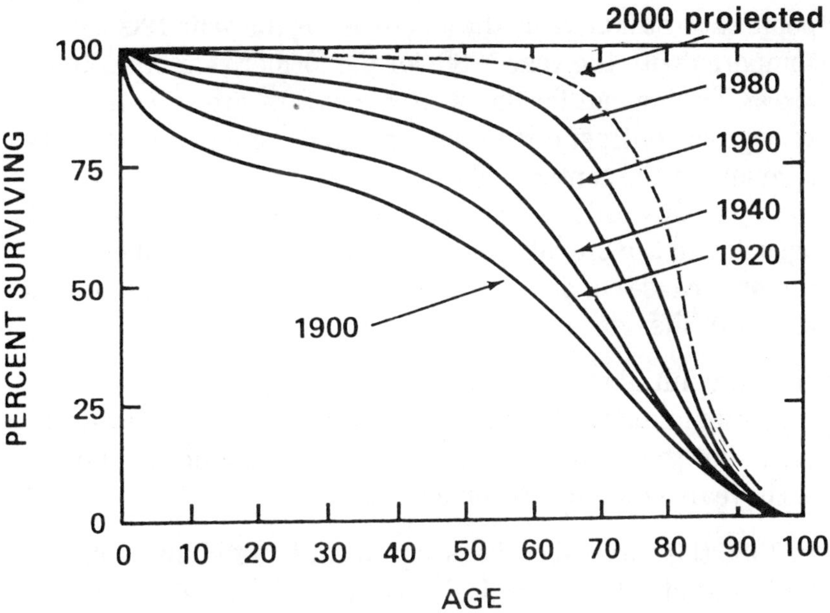

This shows the survival curves for the USA taken from their National Bureau of Health Statistics. The percent of the population that survives to each age for 1900, 1920, 1940, 1960 and 1980 has been plotted against the actual ages shown along the bottom line, and the projected curve for the year 2000 has been added, assuming that present trends continue unaltered – an assumption that may not be justified if social catastrophes overtake us.

Note that all curves meet the bottom line at about age 95 because the percent surviving beyond that age is too small to be shown. How much these curves differ from one another as to where they should meet the bottom line has been debated in the relevant scientific literature, but as the difference is quite small it can be ignored for our purpose.

In order to understand the figure, consider the percent of the population still alive by the age of 60 for the year 1900, compared with the year 1980: for the former year only 50% are still living, but for the latter about 90% are still alive, a very great contrast due to the continual increase in longevity throughout the century. The survival curve for 1900 shows a steady downwards decline because people are dying off at all ages due to the prevalence of infectious diseases and other common causes of death in childhood, adolescence, adulthood, and later life.

Note the initial steep drop for the 1900 curve because of the high rate of mortality in early childhood; no such steep drop occurs for the 1980 curve because death in childhood and the early years of life has become relatively rare.

In 1980 the survival curve is significantly different in shape from that of 1900; instead of a steady decline there is little decline until after the age of about 60, and then there is a steep drop. All the intermediate curves for 1920, 1940 and 1960 are showing this tendency, for progress in health and survival has been continuous during the century. Fries and Crapo, who were mentioned earlier, have pointed out that the curves have become steadily more 'rectangular' in shape and they show what an ideally 'rectangular' curve would be in the figure opposite :

THE RECTANGULAR SURVIVAL CURVE

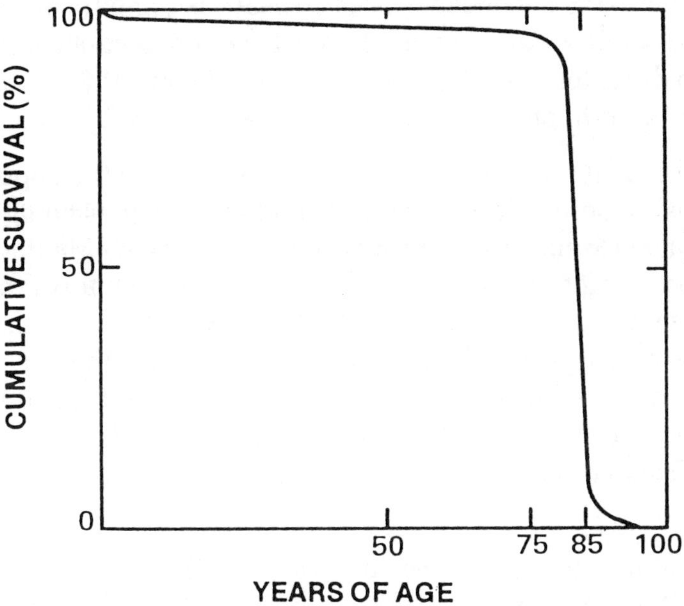

Reproduced from *Vitality and Aging* by J M Fries and L M Crapo with their kind permission and that of their publishers, W H Freeman & Co.

The shape of such a curve would be ideal in that it would indicate a population in which there was very little death below the age of 75; people would live in health and vigour up to an age at which they would drop off their perches quite suddenly.

Earlier, when the concept of the Third Age was explained, the idea of a Fourth Age, as postulated by Peter Laslett, was mentioned. This indicates a period of illness and dependency which can be long or short, and I have questioned whether it is meaningful to refer to it as an 'Age' as some people can and do recover from such a period and revert to the vigour and independence of the Third Age. One of the implications of a rectangular curve is, of course, that any period of dependency prior to death is comparatively brief, and this is what we all long for. It is not the prospect of death itself that is so distasteful to older people, but the fear that they may become sick, unhappy and dependent for a prolonged period.

For some time it has been a common lament that as the population ages so more and more medical and social care is being spent on the older citizens at the expense of the working population. One of the surprising forecasts that can be made from the fact that survival curves are becoming steadily more rectangular is that although there is a steadily increasing proportion of the population entering the Third Age, as they become healthier and spend very little time in any period of final dependency, they will need less and less medical and social care as time goes on if present trends continue.

Sickness and death at all ages due to accidents and inherited defects will always exist, and some people will choose to adopt deleterious life-styles which lead to their premature demise, but it is to be hoped that the great majority of citizens, if educated in sensible ways of conducting their lives and thus preserving their health, will have no significant period of debility and dependence before reaching the end of their natural life-span.

Perhaps there will always be a few remarkable individuals with such a tremendous appetite for life, whatever their state of health, who will say like Zorba in Nikos Kazantzakes' novel *Zorba the Greek* (which was based on an actual individual) 'I've done heaps and heaps of things in my life, but I still did not do enough. Men like me ought to live a thousand years.' The aspirations of such people can never be satisfied.

It goes without saying that this novel concept of the future of the structure and health of the population has not been universally accepted by all modern scientists, and a lively debate continues.

It is understandable that hankering for an ever-continued vigour and health of youth, which has been with us throughout history, was perhaps more evident in former ages when we consider that it is only comparatively recently that the majority of old people have enjoyed a comfortable existence in the later years of their lives.

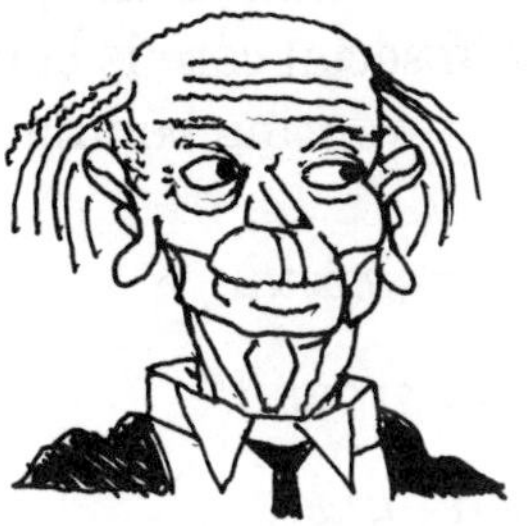

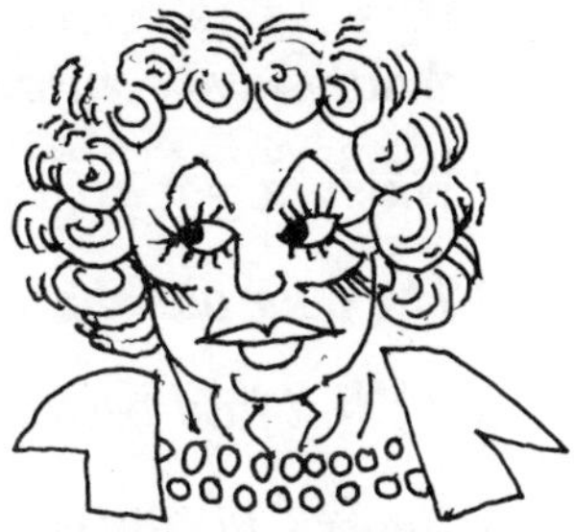

Consider what life must have been like before the days of efficient spectacles, false teeth, hearing-aids and prostheses that we take for granted today. Older people must have lived out their last years in a state of ever-increasing deprivation and misery. To be old was all too often to be pitied by the humane and to be mocked by the heartless.

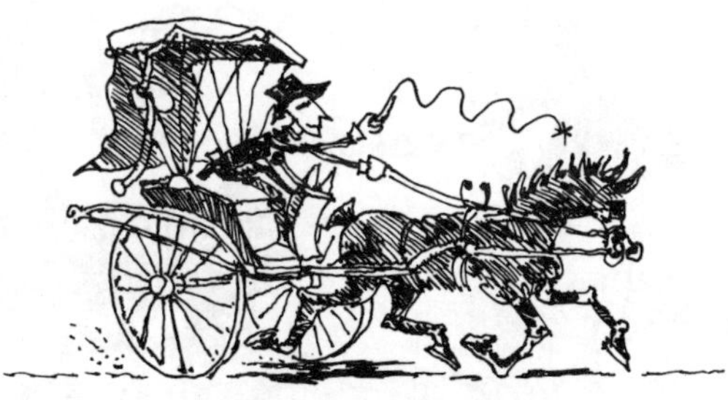

THE FINAL COLLAPSE OF THE ONE-HORSE SHAY

This chapter began with the tale of the wonderful one-horse shay that was carefully constructed out of the very best materials so that each and every part was equally durable, so no one component would wear out before any other. But this vehicle was not any more immortal than are complex living creatures, be they tortoises, mice or human beings, each of which has its limited span. The last verses tell of the final end of the shay which responded to a sudden earthquake shock:

At half past nine by the meet'n'-house clock,
Just the hour of the Earthquake shock!
What do you think the parson found,
When he got up and stared around?
The poor old chaise in a heap or mound
As if it had been to the mill and ground!
You see, of course, if you're not a dunce,
How it went to pieces all at once —
All at once and nothing first —
Just as bubbles do when they burst.

Which is, of course, how we would all like to go – 'All at once and nothing first'.

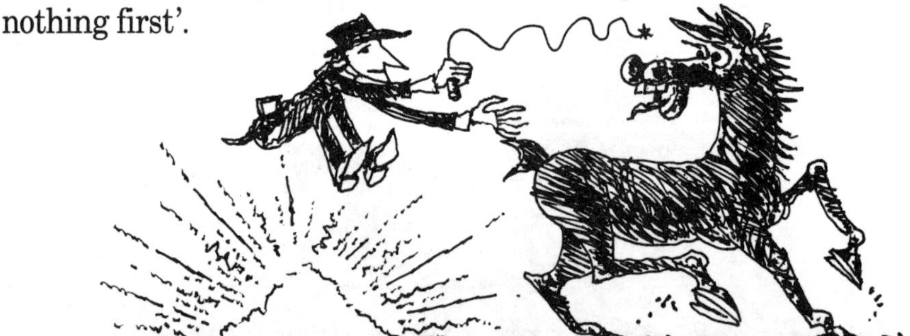

Acceptance of your mortality should make you fully appreciative of the span of years left to you. Nothing can now be done about your genetic make-up which may pre-determine, to some extent, the length of your natural life, nor can the results of accidents and mistakes of past years be fully rectified now. It has been shown, however, the extent to which your present life-style can influence your future health. You may well say with Gratiano in Shakespeare's *Merchant of Venice:*

With mirth and laughter let old wrinkles come;

And let my liver rather heat with wine

Than my heart cool with mortifying groans.

Why should a man whose blood is warm within,

Sit like his grandsire cut in alabaster?

Sleep when he wakes? And creep into the jaundice

By being peevish?

It may be a matter of balancing what is physiologically beneficial for your health against what is psychologically desirable to you: to what degree are you prepared to let your liver 'heat with wine'? Certainly no-one wants to 'creep into a jaundice by being peevish', for that implies becoming depressed, which is one of the greatest ills in later life.

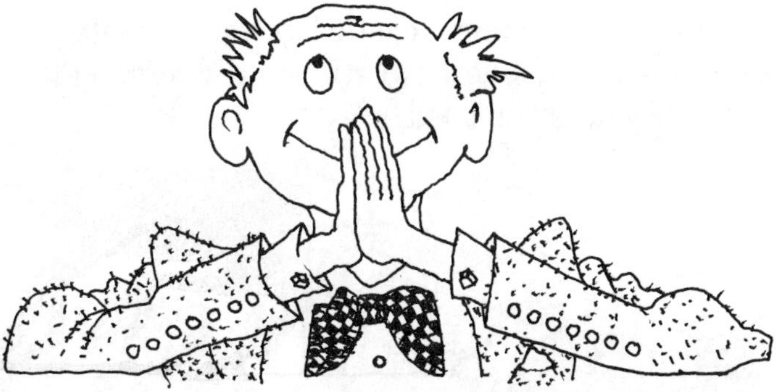

The choice is yours, but it is a choice that is meaningful if you are fully aware of the probable consequences of the life-style that you adopt. There is, of course, the ethical argument that we cannot expect unlimited medical and social help if we are not prepared to act responsibly in looking after ourselves. Self-engendered disability due to unwise indulgence in deleterious habits is expensive for the community at large, so why should they be expected to pay for the folly of the irresponsible few?

Guided by knowledge of sensible health-care, such as I have endeavoured to give in this book, it is up to you to decide how much of anything constitutes 'a little' in applying the maxim 'a little of what you fancy does you good.' Freedom of choice and action is an area of considerable public debate. The public has acquiesced in certain measures of compulsion: we buckle on seat-belts in cars and moderate our drinking before driving, and thus prevent some injury and loss of life, and save hospital casualty departments a great deal of work.

We accept that dangerous drugs should not be freely available over the counter, but on the whole a sensible policy for health-care must depend on individual responsibility plus sensitive support for those unable to make their own choices and arrangements. There may be a danger that some self-declared 'experts' (with or without officially recognized professional qualifications) may have rather stringent standards for you and me and insist that we should be teetotal, rigidly non-smoking, vegetarian, weight-watching, early-rising exercise fanatics, whereas I still stoutly contend that a little of what you fancy does you good.

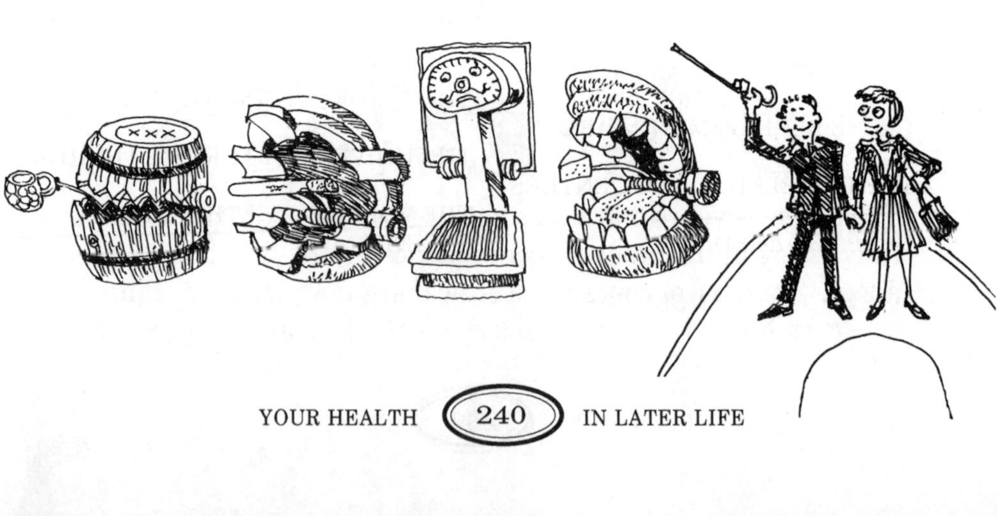

Appendix A

USEFUL ADDRESSES

The organizations in this Appendix:

AGE CONCERN
(four UK main offices)

AGE ACTION IRELAND

ALZHEIMER'S DISEASE SOCIETY

BRITISH ASSOCIATION FOR THE HARD OF HEARING

CANCER LINK

CARERS NATIONAL ASSOCIATION

CENTRE FOR POLICY ON AGEING

THE CONTINENCE ASSOCIATION

CRUSE BEREAVEMENT CARE

THE DISABLED LIVING CENTRES

HELP THE AGED

MARIE CURIE CANCER CARE

NATIONAL ASSOCIATION OF WIDOWS

NATIONAL COUNCIL FOR THE DIVORCED AND SEPARATED

NATIONAL OSTEOPOROSIS SOCIETY

PARKINSON'S DISEASE SOCIETY

THE RAMBLERS ASSOCIATION

THE ROYAL NATIONAL INSTITUTE FOR THE BLIND

THE ROYAL NATIONAL INSTITUTE FOR DEAF PEOPLE

THE STROKE ASSOCIATION

THE UNIVERSITY FOR THE THIRD AGE

THE VOLUNTARY ETHUANASIA SOCIETY

Age Concern England
1268 London Road
London SW16 4EJ
0181 679 8000

Age Concern Scotland
113 Rose Street
Edinburgh EH2 3DT
0131 220 3345

Age Concern Wales
1 Cathedral Road, Cardiff CF1 9SD
01222 371566

Age Concern Northern Ireland
3 Lower Crescent, Belfast BT7 1NR
01232 245 729

Age Concern offers a wide range of services to older people and has numerous groups throughout the UK. Low cost insurance is available to the over 55s. Free Fact Sheets and Briefings are available on receipt of a 9" x 12" sae covering a wide range of topics including: *Dental care in retirement; Help with incontinence; Leisure Education; Disability and Ageing: your rights to social services*; and, *Fitness*.

Age Action Ireland
114 - 116 Pearse Street
Dublin 2 Ireland
+3531 677 9892
A network of providers promoting better policies and services for older people.

Alzheimer's Disease Society
10 Greencoat Place
London SW1P 1PH
0171 306 0606
Provides knowledge about the disease and the aids and services available. They publish a *Newsletter*, a number of factsheets and a guide for people caring for someone with dementia. There are local branches which give support to sufferers and their families

British Association of the Hard of Hearing
7 - 11 Armstrong Road
London W3 7JL
0181 743 1110
Organizes clubs throughout the country for people with all degrees of hearing loss. Some clubs run lip-reading classes.

Cancerlink
11 - 21 Northdown Street
London N1 9BN
0171 833 2818
They provide information and support about all aspects of cancer. There are local groups.

Carers National Association
20 Glasshouse Yard
London EC1
0171 490 8818
They encourage carers to recognize their own needs, develop appropriate support, provide information and advice

and bring such needs to the attention of policy-making bodies.

Centre for Policy on Ageing
25-31 Ironmonger Row
London EC1V 3QP
0171 253 1787
This is an independent organization aiming to raise issues of public importance concerning ageing and old age.

The Continence Foundation
2 Doughty Street
London WC1N 2PH
They sell a range of useful publications and run the Incontinence Information Helpline on 0191 213 0500 (9 - 6 weekdays) for confidential information.

CRUSE Bereavement Care
Cruse house
126 Sheen Road
Richmond,
Surrey TW9 1UR (Helpline)
0181 940 4818 & 0181 332 7227
CRUSE offers help to all bereaved people through counselling, information and social support groups, and have about 200 branches nationwide.

The Disabled Living Centres
Winchester House
11 Cranmer Road
London SW9 6EJ
0171 820 0567
They aim to enable disabled and elderly people to get accurate and impartial information and advice about products designed to help daily living. They can put you in touch with your nearest centre.

Help the Aged
St James' Walk
Clerkenwell Green
London EC1R 0BE
0171 253 0253
They have a Freephone advice and information line (0800 65 00 65) for senior citizens and provide a range of free advice leaflets on health issues, housing, home safety and money matters. They also run residential homes and provide sheltered housing.

Marie Curie Cancer Care
28 Belgrave Square
London SW1X 8QG
0171 235 3325
They provide free medical and nursing care for all who have cancer, and support for their families and carers. Marie Curie Nurses provide care for patients in their own homes throughout the day or night. There are 11 Marie Curie Hospices nationwide.

National Association of Widows
54-57 Allison Street
Digbeth
Birmingham B5 5TH
0121 6543 8348

Advice, information and support is offered to all widows, their families and friends. There are local branches, contact lists and a pen club.

National Council for the Divorced and Separated
PO Box 519
Leicester LEZ 3ZE
0116 2700 595
They are concerned with the interests and welfare divorced and separated people, with 100 branches and 10,000 members nationwide. Inquirers should include a SAE.

National Osteoporosis Society
PO Box 10
Radstock
Bath BA3 3YB
Please send a SAE.
The Society provides advice and information through a national helpline and network of local groups, and raises funds for research

Parkinson's Disease Society
22 Upper Woburn Place
London WC1
0171 383 3513
This society offers information, publications and support on all aspects of Parkinson's Disease. They produce a *Newsletter*, fund research, and have over 220 local branches.

The Ramblers Association
1- 5 Wandsworth Road
London SW8 2XX
0171 582 6878

The Royal National Institute for the Blind
224 Great Portland Street
London W1N 6AA
0171 388 1266
The RNIB provides free information packs and a wide range of services for people suffering from all degrees of visual impairment. Details of your local branch will be supplied on request.

The Royal National Institute for Deaf People
19-23 Featherstone Street
London EC1Y 8SL
0171 296 8000 (Voice)
0171 296 8001 (Text)
The RNID is the largest voluntary organization in the UK representing people with hearing disabilities. They provide information, residential care, training, specialist telephone services, communication support and assistive devices.

The Stroke Association
CHSA House
123-127 Whitecross Street
London EC1Y 8JJ
0171 490 7999
They give help and advice to people who have suffered a stroke and to their families. They offer a Community Service.

The University of the Third Age
26 Harrison Street
London WC1H 8JG
0171 837 8838
There are over 300 local branches and the membership is in excess of 50,000. The primary aim is to provide low-cost educational and social opportunities to people in later life who are no longer in full employment. There are no entrance qualifications and the branches are autonomous, depending on the self-help principle, without the aid of paid tutors.

The Voluntary Euthanasia Society
13 Prince of Wales Terrace
London W8 5PG
0171 937 7770
The Society's principal object is to make it legal for an adult person suffering severe distress from an incurable illness to receive medical help to die at their own considered request. They also issue an advance directive allowing you to reject unwanted and futile treatment which merely prolongs the process of dying.

Appendix B

USEFUL BOOKS

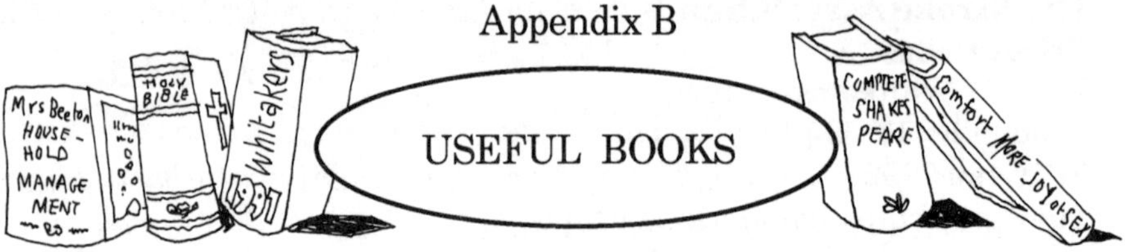

Gerry Bennett (1994) *Alzheimer's Disease and Other Dementias* London: Vermillion.

Pat Blair (1991) *Know Your Medicines.* London: Age Concern.

British Medical Association (1993) *Complementary Medicine* Oxford: Oxford University Press

Jane Brotchie (1995) *Caring for Someone who has Dementia* London: Age Concern.

Alex Comfort (1989) *A Good Age* London: Pan Books.

Philip Coyne and Penny Mares (1995) *Caring for Someone who has a Stroke* London: Age Concern.

Susie Dinan and Dr Craig Sharp (1996) *Fitness for Life* London: from Age Concern, prepared by YMCA, published by Piatkus.

H B Gibson (1995) *On The Tip of Your Tongue: Your Memory in Later Life* London: Third Age Press.

H B Gibson (1997) *Love in Later Life* London: Peter Owen Ltd.

Tony Gibson (1992) *Love, Sex and Power in Later Life* London: Freedom Press.

Margaret Graham (1988) *Keep Moving, Keep Young: Gentle Yoga Exercises for the Elderly* London: Unwin Hyman Ltd.

Wendy and Sally Greengross (1989) *Living, Loving and Ageing* London: Age Concern.

Hamilton Hall (1987) *Be Your Own Back Doctor* London: Grafton Books.

In Touch Publishing (1995) *In Touch Handbook : a comprehensive guide to all the services, benefits and equipment available to blind and partially sighted people* London: In Touch Care Guides

101 Practical Hints for living with poor sight London: In Touch Press

Lorraine Jeffrey (1995) *Hearing Loss and Tinnitus* London: Ward Lock.

Leslie Kenton (1995) *The New Ageless Ageing* London: Arrow Books.

J A Muir Gray and Pat Blair (1990) *Your Health in Retirement* London: Age Concern.

Barbara Robertson (1988) *Fitness for the Over 50s* Wellingborough: Patrick Stephens.

Royal National Institute for the Blind (1994) *You and Your Sight: living with a sight problem* London: RNIB

George Target (1987) *Your Arthritic Hip and You* London: Sheldon Press.

Keith Thompson (1986) *Caring for an Elderly Relative* London: Martin Dunitz.

Richard Villar (1995) *Hip Replacement: A Patient's Guide to Surgery and Recovery* London: Thorsen's Health Series.

Geoffrey Webb and June Copeman (1996) *The Nutrition of Older Adults* London: Edward Arnold.

Fiona van Zwanenberg and Jackie Corder (1990) *Taking Care of Yourself* Bicester: Winslow Press

INDEX

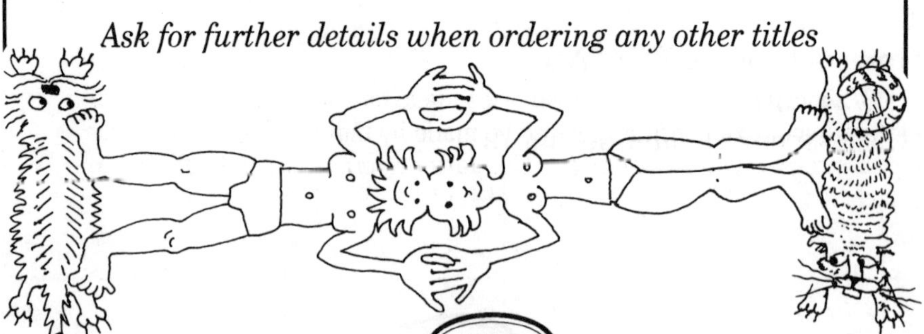

Lifeliners

is a series of booklets that stimulate reflection ~ to see the lines that connect your life not only with the past, but to the present and future as well.

Four titles by Professor Eric Midwinter

Voyage of Rediscovery ~ a guide to writing your life story For individuals or groups wanting to reflect on their lives. (£4.50)

Encore: a guide to planning a celebration of your life ~ it encourages you to think of ways you would like to be remembered by others in the distant future. (£2.50)

The Rhubarb People Eric Midwinter's own *Voyage of Rediscovery*. The author's witty and poignant story of growing up in Manchester in the 1930s. (£4.50)

The Rhubarb People is also available on a 90-minute audio cassette ~ read by the author and including tips on writing your life story. (£5.00)

Getting To Know Me the fourth title by Eric Midwinter ~ is for carers and families of people in care wanting to create a profile of a person ~ their background and relationships, likes and dislikes, as well as the practical information needed to make the caring relationship a positive experience for all concerned. (£4.50)

And . . . by **Enid Irving**

Lifescapes: the landscapes of a lifetime

A *Lifescape* is a collage of memories made for fun or as a very special family heirloom. *Lifescapes* can be made by individuals, in groups, or as an intergenerational activity. This latter approach is particularly recommended for people in care. (£4.50)

Illustrated by Rufus Segar